基础医学实验课程系列教材

Experimental Course of Cell Biology and Medical Genetics

医学细胞与遗传学实验教程

Chinese-English Version

（第二版）

主　审　[美] David Saffen　左　伋

主　编　杨　玲　刘　雯

编写人员　（按姓氏笔画排序）

于文静 (潍坊医学院)

李枚原 (南通大学)

刘　丹 (齐齐哈尔医学院)

刘　雯 (复旦大学)

刘红英 (潍坊医学院)

杨　玲 (复旦大学)

杨　娟 (西安交通大学)

杨云龙 (复旦大学)

吴　丹 (北京大学)

时文涛 (天津医科大学)

贺　颖 (郑州大学)

复旦大学 出版社

前　言
Preface

　　医学是一门实验性或实践性科学。但在传统的医学教育体系中,实验或实践往往是依附于理论课程的,其优点是理论联系实际,符合医学学科的性质;缺点是实验或实践是配合理论,并不自成体系,不能使学生养成通过实验或实践来发现问题、提出问题,进而解决问题的习惯、思维。因此,把实验或实践作为一个独立的课程有一定的意义。在国家提出创新教育的政策下,全国有许多医学院校把实验作为独立的课程开设,如人体功能学实验等。

　　本书是针对部分医学院校独立开设的"细胞与遗传实验"课程编写的教材。本教材从细胞到个体、人群;从正常的细胞结构、遗传物质到细胞损伤的观察与研究、遗传病分析兼顾基础和临床两个方面,涉及细胞与遗传的多种实验技术、方法,并设计了综合性的实验,以开拓学生的实验思路和创新能力。当然,本教材也可作为传统实验课程的指导用书。

　　本教程在编写过程中得到了兄弟院校的大力支持;复旦大学基础医学院细胞与遗传医学系 David Saffen 教授在英文审阅与修改中付出了大量精力;复旦大学基础医学院为教材的出版给予了经费资助;在此一并表示衷心的感谢。由于编者水平有限,在实验内容的选取、方法的描述上都可能有不当之处,敬请读者提出宝贵意见。

杨　玲　刘　雯
2020 年 5 月 1 日

目　　录
Contents

第三篇　遗传的家系和群体分析

Pedigree and population genetic analysis

第四篇　细胞与医学遗传综合实验

Comprehensive projects on cell biology and medical genetics

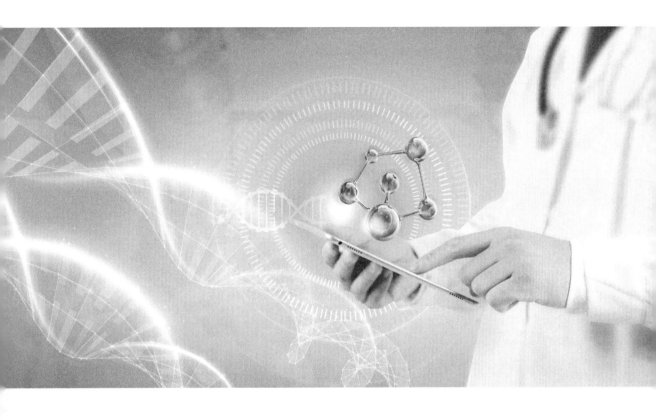

第一篇
组成人体的细胞
Basic experiments in cell biology

第一章　细胞形态的观察

The observation of cell morphology

显微镜扩大了生物学研究的视野。自从 17 世纪人们通过显微镜观察到细胞之后，生物学家利用各种各样的显微镜研究细胞的形态及功能。回顾细胞生物学的历史，可以看出显微镜的不断改良和创新促进了细胞生物学的发展，而这又对显微镜的性能不断提出更高的要求。本章将对几种基本的显微镜技术进行介绍。

Microscopy is central to biological research. Since the 17th century, biologists have used a variety of microscopes to study the morphology and function of cells. The field of microscopy has revolutionized our understanding of cell biology and the development of cell biology has repeatedly set higher requirements for the performance of microscopes. This chapter introduces several fundamental types of microscopy.

第一节 ◎ 光学显微镜技术

Light microscopy

在细胞学研究中，光学显微镜技术发挥了重要作用。目前，人们将多种现代生物学技术、计算机技术融入光学显微镜技术，使光学显微镜能显示出更细微、更清晰的细胞结构。

Light microscope (LM) plays a critical role in modern cell biology.

一、普通光学显微镜技术　Bright-field microscopy

光学显微镜一般由光学部分、机械部分和照明部分组成。其中光学部分最为关键，它由目镜(eyepiece)、物镜(objective lens)组成。普通光学显微镜的最大分辨率为 $0.2~\mu m$。由于动物细胞一般是无色与半透明的，所以样品在观察前要经过染色。不同的染料对某种细胞组分有特异的吸附，这样便能形成足够的反差以区分该种细胞组分。如最常用的染色液苏木精对带负电荷的分子有较强亲和力，因此可揭示出 DNA、RNA 和酸性蛋白质在细胞中的分布；而伊红和亚甲蓝能特异性地与不同蛋白结合，从而显示出这些蛋白在细胞内的分布情况。

Bright-field microscope is an instrument that uses visible light and magnifying lenses to examine small objects. Most bright-field microscopes use two lenses (objective lens and eyepiece) to produce a magnified image. In bright-field microscopy, the light source and lens are placed on opposite sides of the sample, and images are produced based on how the sample absorbs, scatters, or deflects the light passing through it. The maximum resolution of light microscope is 0.2 μm.

二、相差和微分干涉相差显微镜技术　Phase contrast and differential interference contrast microscopy

1932 年,荷兰物理学家 Fritz Zernike 研究发现光线在通过生物标本时,除了波长和振幅的变化外,还有相位的差异,只有将这种相位差转变成振幅差时,才能被人眼分辨出来,即相差理论。他将这一理论应用于显微镜,从而发明了相差显微镜(phase contrast microscope)。微分干涉相差显微镜(differential interference contrast microscope)是基于相差技术而发明的,能够显示结构的三维立体投影影像。相差和微分干涉相差显微镜是对透明标本能够产生高对比度图像的互补技术,因此观察样品不需要进行染色处理。在细胞生物学实验中,常用的是倒置相差显微镜,它的光源和聚光镜装在载物台上方,相差物镜在载物台下方,这样更便于观察培养瓶中的活细胞。

Different types of microscopes have been developed to improve resolution and contrast of the sample. Phase contrast microscopy, first described in 1932 by the Dutch physicist Frits Zernike, is a contrast-enhancing optical technique that can be utilized to produce high-contrast images of transparent specimens. With phase contrast microscopy, the living cells can be examined in their natural state without previously being stained.

Phase contrast and differential interference contrast (DIC) microscopy are complementary techniques capable of producing high-contrast images of transparent biological phases. The inverted phase-contrast microscope is often used in biological experiments, since it can be used to study living cells (usually in culture).

三、荧光显微镜技术　Fluorescence microscopy

荧光显微镜是通过一定波长的光激发样品,进而产生特定波长和颜色的荧光,用来观察和分辨某些细胞组分和生物大分子的一种显微镜。

细胞本身存在的物质经紫外线照射后发出的荧光称自发荧光。另一些细胞内成分经紫外线照射后不发荧光,但若用荧光染料进行染色后,就能在荧光显微镜下显示荧光,这种荧光称为继发荧光。目前,可供选择的荧光染料非常多,如异硫氰酸荧光素(FITC)、藻红蛋白(PE)、碘化丙啶(PI)、联脒基苯吲哚(DAPI)和 Hoechest 33258 等。免疫细胞化学检测,可以通过荧光染料标记的抗体和相应的抗原结合形成抗原抗体复合物,在荧光显微镜下经特定波长激光激发后发射荧光,从而观察抗原的有无、多少以及细胞内的分布。

A fluorescence microscope is an optical microscope that uses fluorescence to study and distinguish certain cellular components and biomacromolecules. The specimen is illuminated with light of a specific wavelength which is absorbed by the fluorescent dyes. Fluorescent dyes, also termed fluorophores. FITC(fluorescein isothiocyanate), PE (phycoerythrin), PI (propidium iodide), 4′,6-diamidino-2-phenylindole (DAPI), and Hoechst 33258 are among the most widely used fluorescent dyes.

四、激光扫描共聚焦显微镜技术 Laser scanning confocal microscopy

激光扫描共聚焦显微镜是在荧光显微镜成像的基础上,通过针孔排除非焦平面及焦平面非焦点光斑信息,获取样品的"光切片"图像,通过计算机重构,得到细胞、亚细胞器或生物大分子的结构或组织分布。这样形成的图像异常清晰,其分辨率比普通荧光显微镜提高1.4～1.7倍。激光扫描共聚焦显微镜的工作原理见图1-1。图1-1A中显示激光束(光源,laser)经入射小孔(light source pinhole)被二向色镜(dichroic mirror)反射后,通过显微物镜(objective lens)汇聚到待观察的标本(specimen)内部某一焦点(focal point)处。图1-1B中显示经激光照射后,从焦点发出的荧光(fluorescence light),被物镜重新收集后通过二向色镜并透过出射小孔(detection pinhole)到达光电探测器(detector),变成电信号后送入计算机。而残余的激光则被二向色镜反射,不会被探测到。通过分层聚焦后,将获得的分层图像进行三维重建,进而分析样品的形态和荧光强度等特征。

Laser scanning confocal microscopes are based on fluorescence microscopy. They employ a pair of pinhole apertures to limit the specimen focal plane to a confined volume approximately a micron in size. Fig. 1-1 shows the principle of laser scanning confocal microscopy. Fig. 1-1A shows that laser beams are reflected by dichroic mirror through the confocal pinhole and are aggregated through the objective lens and then focused onto a focal point inside the specimens. Fig. 1-1B shows that the fluorescence produced by exposure to the laser is recollected by the objective and sent directly through the dichroic mirror and detection pinhole to the detector and fed into a computer.

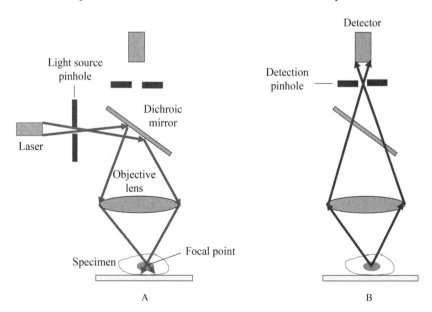

图1-1 激光共焦点扫描显微镜的原理
Fig. 1-1 Principle of laser scanning confocal microscope

五、显微镜的基本使用方法　Use of microscopes

放置显微镜于实验台上;将玻片放置于载物台上,用推片器弹簧夹夹住,将所要观察的部位调节到通光孔的正中;通过粗调节器将载物台降至最低,转动转换器,将最低倍数的物镜对准样品;使用粗调节器获得大概的物像,并使用细调节器直到视野中出现清晰的物像为止;转动转换器,调换上高倍镜头,通过细调节器获得清晰的物像;如果没有观察到想要的图像,则需要重新调回至低倍镜,并重新聚焦。

Set the microscope on a stable table and plug it into a nearby outlet. Place the slide on the microscope stage with the center of the slide over the hole through which the light will pass. Clip the slide onto the stage with the stage clips and turn on the microscope. Turn the coarse focus knob to lower the stage as far as possible and turn the microscope's lenses so the shortest one，which is the lowest magnification，is pointing down. Look through the eyepiece and turn the rough focus knob to obtain a general focus. Use the fine adjustment knob to obtain a clear focus. Without any further adjustments，switch the objective lens to the next highest magnification then focus using the fine adjustment. If you cannot see the specimen at this point，go back to low power and re-centre and refocus it.

第二节 ◎ 电子显微镜技术
Electron microscopy

电子显微镜能够观察到更细微的结构,在生物学研究中,常被用于组织、细胞、细胞器以及生物大分子的观察。

Electron microscopy（EM）is a technique for obtaining high resolution images of specimens. In biological research，EM used to investigate the detailed structure of tissues，cells，organelles and macromolecular complexes.

一、透射电子显微镜技术　Transmission electron microscopy

(一)基本原理与结构　Basic principle and components

1933 年,Ruska 发明了以电子束为光源的透射电子显微镜（transmission electron microscope，TEM）。电子束穿透超薄样品时,会和样品中的原子发生散射,进而形成图像。电子束的波长要比可见光和紫外光短得多,并且电子束的波长与发射电子束的电压平方根成反比,也就是说电压越高,波长越短,分辨率更高。普通的 TEM 分辨率可达 0.2 nm,像球差校正透射电子显微镜（spherical aberration corrected transmission electron microscope，ACTEM）的分辨率甚至可以达到 0.06 nm。

Transmission electron microscopy（TEM） also named conventional TEM（CTEM） employs a close-to-parallel electron beam transmitted through a specimen to form an image. TEM is used to reveal the ultrastructure of cells.

透射电子显微镜主要由 4 部分组成(图 1 - 2)。①电子束照明系统:包括电子枪、聚光镜。由高频电流加热钨丝发出电子,经高压使电子加速,经过聚光镜汇聚成电子束。②成像系统:包括物镜、中间镜与投影镜等。它们是若干精密加工的中空圆柱体,里面装置线圈,通过改变线圈的电流大小,调节圆柱体空间的磁场强度。电子束经过磁场时发生螺旋式运动,最终的结果如同光线通过玻璃透镜时一样,聚焦成像。③真空系统:用两级真空泵不断抽气,保持电子枪、镜筒及记录系统内的高真空。④记录系统:电子成像须通过荧光屏显示用于观察,或用感光胶片记录下来。

TEM consists of the following main components (Fig. 1 - 2). ①Electron gun:after connecting to a high-voltage source of about $100 \sim 300$ kV, the electron gun releases electrons by either thermionic or field electron emission into a vacuum. ②Electromagnetic lenses:the electromagnetic lenses consist of coils. An electromagnetic field is created when an electric current is passed through these coils. ③Vacuum system: electrons behave like light when passing through a vaccum. Different vacuum pumps are used to obtain and maintain a high vacuum. ④Image viewing and recording system.

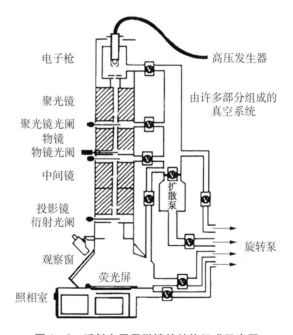

图 1 - 2 透射电子显微镜的结构组成示意图

Fig. 1 - 2 Components and structure of transmission electron microscopy

由于电子在空气里穿透力很弱,所以电子显微镜的镜筒必须抽成真空,否则高速运动的电子和气体分子相互碰撞,会使高速电子散射而偏离轨道,使电子显微镜不能正常工作。电子显微镜镜筒的真空度越高,其使用性能也就越好。

透射电子显微镜可以提取的样本信息主要依赖于 4 个参数:显微镜的分辨率、电子束的能量扩散、标本的厚度和标本的组成及稳定性。

The information extracted by TEM depends critically on four parameters:resolution of the microscope，energy spread of the electron beam，thickness of the specimen and composition and stability of the specimen.

(二) 电子显微镜制样技术　Sample preparation for transmission electron microscopy

1. 固定　Fixation

固定是电子显微镜样品制备过程中最重要的一个环节,若固定方法选得适当,样品的超微结构将尽可能接近活体状态。目前常用的固定剂为四氧化锇(OsO_4)和戊二醛等。组织可以通过浸没或灌注来固定。最常用的方法是浸入式。根据固定的组织标本不同,固定所需时间是可变的,通常 4℃固定 4 h 或者过夜。

Fixation is a critical step. The sample should be fixed in a way that the ultrastructure of the cells or tissues remain as close to the living material as possible. Osmium tetroxide and glutaraldehyde are fixatives used in TSM. Fixation can be achieved by perfusion or immersion. The most often used method is immersion. Fixation time is variable，depending on tissue，but is usually from 4 hours to overnight at 4℃.

2. 脱水　Dehydration

固定后,样品通过丙酮或系列梯度乙醇脱水。脱水的时间取决于样品的大小和种类。

After fixation，the sample is dehydrated through a series of increasing concentrations of acetone or ethanol. The dehydration times should be adjusted according to size and kind of tissue.

3. 包埋　Embedding

包埋的目的是要使样品中各种细微结构在切片中得到均匀良好的支撑,使切成的超薄切片仍能保持连续完整,并且有足够的强度,可耐受干燥以及电子轰击、高温和真空挥发。

The purpose of embedding is to provide tissues with enough firmness to permit the cutting of thin sections.

4. 切片　Sectioning

由于电子束的穿透能力有限,为了获得较高分辨率,需要制成厚度仅为 40～50 nm 的超薄切片。包埋好的组织用超薄切片机切成超薄切片,以热膨胀或螺旋推进的方式推进样品切片。

After embedding，tissue needs to be cut into ultra-thin slices (40 to 50 nm).

5. 染色　Staining

由于生物样品多是由 C、H、O、N 等元素组成,这些元素原子序数低,散射电子能力弱,在电子显微镜下的反差很弱。因此,通常需用高分子量的金属盐对超薄切片进行染色,以形成明暗反差。目前,常采用双重染色法,即先用铀染液染色,再用铅染液染色。

Staining is used to enhance contrast in tissues. Heavy metal salts are always used for staining in electron microscopy.

(三) 负染色技术　Negative staining

一些细小的颗粒标本如线粒体基粒、核糖体、纤维蛋白、病毒等可以通过负染色(negative stain)电子显微镜技术观察其精细结构,其分辨率可达 1.5 nm 左右。负染色电子显微镜技术中,染料与样品结合后包裹在样品周围,当电子束通过样品时,背景呈深色,而样品呈白色。常用的染色剂如 2% 磷钨酸水溶液等。

Negative staining is always applied in transmission electron microscopy. In this technique, the background is stained, instead of the actual specimen, allowing small objects such as mitochondria, ribosomes, fibrin, viruses and bacteria to be clearly observed.

二、扫描电子显微镜技术　Scanning electron microscope

20 世纪 60 年代扫描电子显微镜(scanning electron microscope，SEM)逐渐引起人们的重视,其电子枪发射出的电子束被电磁透镜汇聚成极细的电子"探针",在样品表面进行"扫描",电子束可激发样品表面放出二次电子,二次电子产生的多少与样品的形状有关。二次电子由探测器收集,并被转化成光信号,再经光电倍增管和放大器转变成电压信号来控制荧光屏上电子束的强度。这样,样品不同部位上产生二次电子多或少的差异,直接反映在荧光屏相应部位亮或暗的差别,从而得到一幅放大的立体很强的图像。

Scanning electron microscope (SEM) is one type of electron microscope，which uses a focused beam of electrons to produce images of samples through scanning the surface of samples. In the scanning electron microscope，the narrow incident electron beam interact with the specimen surface，then produce secondary electrons，backscattered electrons，and characteristic X-rays. All the signals are collected by one or more detectors to form images. Images are displayed on the computer screen.

（杨　玲）

第二章　细胞培养

Cell culture

　　细胞是构成生命有机体的基本单位,也是研究一切生命现象及其本质的基本材料。人体是由多细胞构成的整体,在整体条件下研究单个细胞或某一群细胞在体内(*in vivo*)的功能活动是十分困难的。如果把活细胞拿到体外(*in vitro*)进行培养、观察和研究,则要方便得多。活细胞离体后于模拟体内生理环境等特定的体外条件下,进行孵育培养使之生存、增殖并进行生理活动的过程就称为细胞培养(cell culture)或细胞培养技术(cell culture technique)。细胞培养广泛应用于细胞工程、肿瘤、免疫学以及体细胞遗传等研究领域。

　　The cell is the basic unit which makes up all living organisms and is the basic experimental material used to explore the phenomenon of life. The human body is composed of many kinds of cells. It is often difficult to study the functions of groups of cells *in vivo*. In such cases, it is more convenient to study living cells *in vitro*: that is by culturing living cells under conditions that allow them to proliferate and carry out normal physiological activities. Cell culture is widely used in biological research, including studies in the fields of bioengineering, cancer and immunology.

第一节 ◎ 细胞培养概述
Overview of cell culture

　　细胞培养是指从机体内的组织中取出细胞,在体外模拟体内的生理条件,使之生存、生长、繁殖,并维持其结构和功能的培养技术。

　　Cell culture refers to techniques that allow cells isolated from tissues *in vivo* to grow, reproduce, and maintain their structures and functions under simulated physiological conditions *in vitro*.

一、细胞培养的条件　cell culture conditions

　　人工模拟环境是否与体内生理环境一致决定了细胞在体外能否生存以及生活质量的好坏。概括说来,这种人工模拟的生存环境应主要包括:营养需求、温度、渗透压、酸碱度(pH)以及有无污染等几方面因素。

　　The production of artificial environments consistent with physiological environments determines whether cells can survive and function normally. At very least，simulated environments must provide cells with appropriate nutrition，temperature，osmotic pressure，pH and removal of metabolic waste.

（一）营养需求　Nutrition

体外培养细胞时,营养需求是满足其生存、生长及增殖的首要条件。细胞培养基就是在体外培养细胞时供给细胞营养和促使细胞生长增殖的基础物质。

Appropriate nutrition is the primary requirement for the cells to survive，grow and proliferate *in vitro*. The culture medium is the basic source of nutrition and substances that promote cell growth and proliferation.

1. 细胞对营养的需求　The nutritional requirements for cells

离体培养细胞对营养的需求基本上与体内相同,主要包括氨基酸、糖类、无机盐类、维生素、蛋白质、脂类和微量元素等几个方面。

The nutritional requirements for cells *in vitro* are basically the same as those *in vivo*，comprising mainly amino acids，saccharides，inorganic salts，vitamins，proteins，lipids and trace elements.

（1）氨基酸 Amino acids：氨基酸既是细胞合成蛋白质的原料,也是细胞重要的能量来源。氨基酸的种类及数量影响着细胞的密度、增殖和活力等诸多方面。几乎所有的细胞均需要下列12种氨基酸:精氨酸、缬氨酸、酪氨酸、组氨酸、色氨酸、苏氨酸、苯丙氨酸、蛋氨酸、赖氨酸、亮氨酸、异亮氨酸和胱氨酸。

Amino acids are not only the raw materials for protein synthesis，but also important sources of energy for cells. The density，proliferation and vitality of cells can be affected by kinds and amount of amino acids. Almost all cells require the following 12 amino acids：arginine，valine，tyrosine，histidine，tryptophan，threonine，phenylalanine，methionine，lysine，leucine，isoleucine and cystine.

（2）糖类 Saccharides：糖类物质是细胞最主要的能量来源,也是生物合成核酸、氨基酸、脂类物质的重要碳源。用于细胞培养的糖类物质主要有葡萄糖和半乳糖,其中以葡萄糖最为常用。

Saccharides are the most important energy source for cells and are also important sources of carbon for the biosynthesis of nucleic acids，amino acids and lipids. Glucose and galactose are the main sugars used in cell culture，of which glucose is the most often used.

（3）无机盐 Inorganic salts：无机盐对基础培养基渗透压的调节具有重要作用,同时还可调节细胞跨膜电位、细胞附着以及一些酶的活性等。经常添加的无机盐离子主要有钠、钾、镁、磷、钙等。

Inorganic salts play an important role in regulating the osmotic pressure of culture media. In addition，specific inorganic ions regulate transmembrane potentials，cell adhesion and the activity of enzymes. The inorganic ions most often included in culture media include sodium，potassium，magnesium，phosphorus and calcium.

(4) 维生素 Vitamins：维生素是诸多细胞代谢活动重要的辅酶,对细胞的活力与增殖具有较大的影响。生物素、叶酸、烟酰胺、维生素 B_2(核黄素)、维生素 C、维生素 B_{12}、吡哆醇等都是培养基需要添加的成分,尤以 B 族维生素最为常见。

Vitamins function as coenzymes in many essential metabolic pathways, and therefore greatly influence cell vitality and proliferation. Vitamins that often need to be added to culture medium, include biotin, folic acid, nicotinamide, vitamin B_2 (riboflavin), vitamin C, vitamin B_{12}, and pyridoxine, with B vitamins the most often added.

(5) 脂类 Lipids：脂肪酸和脂类物质是某些特定细胞系的必需成分。例如：用于培养胆固醇依赖的杂交瘤的培养基就需要添加一定量胆固醇。

Fatty acids and lipids are usually supplied by serum and are essential for certain cell lines. For example, sufficient amounts of cholesterol must be included in medium used to cultivate cholesterol-dependent hybridomas.

(6) 微量元素 Trace elements：微量元素常被添加入无血清培养基,以弥补因未添加血清所造成的微量元素缺失或不足。主要有锌、铜、硒等,其中硒对于清除培养基中由代谢产生的自由基具有重要作用。

Trace elements, including zinc, copper, and selenium, are often added to serum-free medium. Selenium, for example, plays an important role in the scavenging of highly reactive free radicals released from cells into the culture medium.

2. 培养基　Culture medium

用于细胞培养的培养基种类繁多,按其来源分为天然培养基和合成培养基两类。在细胞培养技术发展的早期,所用的细胞培养基多是来自于淋巴液、血浆、血清以及各种组织提取液,常被称为天然培养基。目前使用最普遍的天然培养基是血清。血清是一种极其复杂的混合物,包含大量蛋白以及多种生长因子、激素、氨基酸、糖、胰蛋白酶抑制剂、脂类物质、无机盐、微量元素等。最常用的血清主要有胎牛血清(fetal bovine serum,FBS)、新生牛血清(newborn calf serum,NCS)和小牛血清(calf serum,CS)等。目前,这种天然的培养基常被作为添加剂与合成培养基合用,常见的血清添加比例为 5%～20%。合成培养基是根据细胞所需物质的种类和数量严格配制而成的培养基,包括碳水化合物、氨基酸、脂类、无机盐、维生素、微量元素和细胞生长因子等。

There are many kinds of medium used for cell culture. These can be roughly divided into natural culture medium and synthetic culture medium, depending upon their source. In the early stages of cell culture techniques, natural media derived from lymph, plasma, serum, and various tissue extracts were often used. Currently, most natural medium contains serum, such as fetal bovine serum, newborn bovine serum and calf serum. This natural medium is usually used as an additive to synthetic medium at concentration of 5% to 20%. Culture medium is strictly formulated according to the kinds and quantities of substances required by specific types of cells. Components include carbohydrates, amino acids, lipids, inorganic salts, vitamins, trace elements, and cell growth factors.

（二）温度　Temperature

体外培养的细胞需要在一定的温度条件下才能存活，不同细胞适宜的培养温度与细胞的物种来源有关。例如，哺乳类动物细胞包括人类细胞的理想培养温度多在 $36\sim37℃$；鸟类细胞适宜的培养温度在 $38.5℃$；昆虫细胞的培养温度在 $25℃$；冷血脊椎动物的培养温度在 $18\sim25℃$。

Cells cultured *in vitro* need appropriate temperatures to survive. The suitable temperature for different cells is related to the species of animals from which they were isolated. For example, the optimum culture temperature for mammals, including human cells, is 36 to 37℃, for bird cells 38.5℃, insect cells 25℃ and cold-blooded vertebrates 18 to 25℃.

不适合的培养温度会严重影响细胞的存活及生长状态。通常，细胞对低温具有较长时间的耐受性，甚至可在低于适宜温度的一定范围内生长。但如果培养温度高于适宜温度时（如在 $39℃$ 条件下培养人类细胞），细胞常会在几小时内死亡。因此，定期检查细胞培养箱的温度非常重要。

Inappropriate culture temperatures will seriously affect the survival and growth of cells. Usually, cells can tolerant low temperatures for a long time and can even grow in a certain range below their optimal temperature. However, if the culture temperature is higher than the appropriate temperature, example, human cells cultured at 39℃, the cells will often die within a few hours. Therefore, it is very important to regularly check the temperature of cell culture incubators.

（三）渗透压　Osmotic pressure

离体的细胞必须生长在等渗的液体环境中才能维持细胞的正常形态、结构，并有助于细胞对物质运输的调控。渗透压的大小主要由培养基中各种盐成分的浓度决定。适宜的渗透压因细胞的种类及物种来源不同而异。例如，培养人类细胞的理想渗透压为 290 mmol/kg；培养大多数哺乳类动物细胞的理想渗透压多在 $260\sim320$ mmol/kg；培养小鼠细胞的理想渗透压多在 320 mmol/kg 左右。大多数细胞对渗透压都有一定的耐受性。

In vitro, cells must be cultivated in an isotonic liquid environment to maintain their normal morphology and structure and maintain normal trans-membrane transport of ions and other solutes. Osmotic pressure is determined primarily by the concentrations of various salts in the medium. The appropriate osmotic pressure varies with the cell type and species of origin. For example, the ideal osmotic pressure for culturing most mammalian cells is in the range from 260 to 320 mmol/kg, with cultured human cells at 290 mmol/kg and cultured mouse cells at 320 mmol/kg. Most cells, however, are tolerant to small changes in osmotic pressure.

（四）气相和酸碱度　Gaseous phase and pH

体外培养的细胞对气体环境也有一定的要求。多数细胞在培养时需要氧气的存在，但氧分压多维持在略低于大气中的氧分压的水平，因为过高的氧分压会造成细胞的损伤。二氧化碳（CO_2）也是细胞培养所需要的，其与培养基酸碱度（pH）的维持密切相关，CO_2 浓度的升高会引起培养基 pH 值的降低。体外培养细胞时的气体环境常由 95% 的空气和 5% 的 CO_2 构成,针对培养对象和培养基缓冲系统的不同,CO_2 的浓度常在 2%～10% 之间变化。

Cells cultured *in vitro* also have specific requirements for the composition of their gas environment. Cells need oxygen to grow in culture. The partial pressure of oxygen is maintained at a level slightly lower than that of oxygen in the atmosphere, however, because excessive partial pressure of oxygen can cause cell damage. CO_2 is also needed for cell culture to maintain the optimal medium pH. Increasing the concentration of CO_2 will cause pH of the medium to decrease. When culturing cells *in vitro*, the gas environment is usually composed of 95% air and 5% CO_2. The concentration of CO_2 varies from 2% to 10% according the cell type and medium buffering system.

适宜大多数细胞生长的培养基 pH 多维持在 7.0～7.4,而细胞在培养过程中所释放出的代谢产物尤其是 CO_2 会造成培养基 pH 值的迅速下降,非常不利于细胞的继续生长。为了尽可能长时间的将培养基的 pH 值稳定在适当范围,常借助 CO_2 -碳酸氢盐缓冲体系或有机缓冲体系(如 HEPES 缓冲液)来解决这一问题。

The culture medium pH range for most cells is maintained 7.0 to 7.4. Metabolites released by cells during the culture, especially CO_2, can cause a rapid decline of the pH of the medium, which is often detrimental to the continued growth of cells. To maintain the pH of the culture medium in an appropriate range for as long as possible, CO_2-bicarbonate buffer system or organic buffer system (such as HEPES solution) are often used.

(五) 无污染环境　Non-polluted environment

细菌等微生物的污染,以及不同细胞间的交叉污染也是细胞培养时必须要避免的事情。可通过严格的过滤除菌或灭菌处理,并使用抗生素来降低污染的发生概率。在细胞培养中最常使用的抗生素是青霉素(常用浓度是 25～100 μg/ml)与链霉素(25～100 μg/ml)。

In addition to toxic chemicals, microbial contamination by micoplasma, bacteria or yeasts, as well as cross-contamination between different cell types must be avoided in cell culture. The probability of contamination can be reduced by strict filtration and sterilization protocol and the use of antibiotics. The most commonly used antibiotics in cell culture are penicillin (25～100 μg/ml) and streptomycin (25～100 μg/ml).

因此,细胞培养所需的一切器皿、试剂、实验材料等都要严格按规范进行刷洗、消毒。无菌操作的严格执行也是细胞培养成功的关键。

All the petri dishes, reagents, and experimental materials required for cell culture must be strictly disinfected and sterilized according to the laboratory specifications. Strict aseptic manipulation is also a key to the success of cell culture.

二、无菌操作 Sterile cell culture

（一）无菌室的灭菌 Sterilization of aseptic culture rooms

1. 定期打扫无菌室 Regularly cleaning of aseptic culture rooms

每周打扫一次，先用自来水拖地、擦桌子、超净工作台等，然后用 3‰甲酚（来苏尔）或者苯扎溴铵（新洁尔灭）或者 0.5%过氧乙酸擦拭。

Once a week：mop the floor，clean the tables and laminar flow cabinets，first with water and then with either cresol（Lysol，3‰），benzalkonium bromide（neogeramine，3‰）or peroxyacetic acid（0.5%）.

2. 细胞培养箱灭菌 Sterilization of cell culture incubator

先用 3‰苯扎溴铵（新洁尔灭）擦拭，然后用 75%乙醇或者 0.5%过氧乙酸擦拭，再用紫外灯照射灭菌。

First，wipe the incubator with benzalkonium bromide（neogeramine，3‰），then with ethanol（75%）or peroxyacetic acid（0.5%）. Finally，irradiate it with ultraviolet light.

3. 实验前灭菌 Sterilization before experiments

打开紫外灯、臭氧杀菌机和空气净化器系统各 20～30 min。

Turn on the ultraviolet lamp，trioxide sterilizer，and air purifier system for 20 to 30 min each.

4. 实验后灭菌 Sterilization after experiments

用 75%乙醇（3‰苯扎溴铵）擦拭超净台和实验台等。

Use ethanol（75%）or benzalkonium bromide（bromogeramine，3‰）to wipe the laminar flow cabinet and laboratory benches.

（二）实验人员的无菌准备 Aseptic protocol for laboratory personnel

（1）用肥皂洗手。

Wash hands with soap.

（2）穿好隔离衣、戴好隔离帽、口罩，换上拖鞋。

Wear isolation clothes，hats，masks and put on slippers.

（3）用 75%乙醇棉球擦净双手。

Clean hands with 75% ethanol cotton ball.

（三）注意事项 Notes

（1）凡是带入超净工作台内的物品均要用 75%乙醇擦拭外表面。

All the items brought into the laminar flow cabinet should be wiped with 75% ethanol on the outside.

（2）吸取两种以上的使用液时要注意更换吸管，防止交叉污染。

When pipetting more than two kinds of liquids，attention should be paid to replacing pipettes to prevent cross-contamination.

（3）在对不同细胞进行操作时应避免使用同一瓶培养基或使用同一个吸管。

Avoid using the same medium or pipette when handling different cells.

第二节 ◎ 培养细胞的生物学特性
Biological characteristics of cultured cells

一、体外培养细胞的分型 Classification of cultured cells *in vitro*

体外培养细胞时，主要有两种培养体系：一种是贴附依赖型，一种是悬浮型。

When culturing cells *in vitro*, there are two main culture systems: attachment-dependent and suspension-dependent.

（一）贴附依赖型 Attachment-dependent type

大多数培养细胞贴附生长，属于贴附依赖型细胞，依据培养细胞在体外的形态大致可将其分为以下 4 种类型。

Most cultured cells display adherent growth and are attachment-dependent cells. Based on morphology, cultured cells *in vitro* can be roughly divided into the following four types.

1. 上皮细胞型 Epithelium cell type

细胞多呈扁平不规则多角形，中央有圆形细胞核，细胞彼此紧密相连成单层膜。此型细胞多起源于内、外胚层的细胞，如皮肤表皮及其衍生物、消化管上皮、肝、胰、肺泡上皮等。来源于人类胚肾的 HEK293 细胞、来源于人类肝脏组织的 HEPG2 细胞、来源于人类子宫颈的 HeLa 细胞就属此类。

Most of the cells are flat and with irregular polygonal cell bodies and round nuclei in their centers. These cell form closely linked monolayers at high culture densities. Most of these cells originate from endodermal or ectodermal cells, such as skin epidermis and derivatives, digestive tract epithelium, hepatopancreas and alveolar epithelium. HEK293 cells from human embryonic kidney, HEPG2 cells from human liver tissue and HeLa cells from human cervix belong to this category.

2. 成纤维细胞型 Fibroblast cell type

胞体多呈梭形或不规则三角形，中央有卵圆形细胞核，呈放射状生长。除真正的成纤维细胞外，起源于中胚层间充质组织的心肌、平滑肌、成骨细胞、血管内皮等均呈此型形态。另外，也常将一些与成纤维细胞形态类似的培养细胞归为此类，如源自小鼠胚胎的 NIH 3T3、小鼠结缔组织的 L929、中国仓鼠卵巢的 CHO、叙利亚地鼠肾脏的 BHK - 21 等。

Cell bodies are mostly spindle-shaped or form irregular triangles, with oval nuclei in the center and display radial growth. In addition to actual fibroblasts, cells derived from myocardium, smooth muscle, osteoblasts or vascular endothelium originating from mesodermal mesenchymal tissue all show this pattern. In addition, some cultured cells with similar fibroblast morphology are often classified as this type, including NIH 3T3 from mouse embryos, L929 from mouse connective tissue, CHO from Chinese hamster ovaries, BHK - 21 from Syrian hamster kidneys.

3. 游走细胞型 Migratory cell type

多呈散在生长,一般不连成片,具有活跃的游走或变形运动能力,且方向不确定。此型细胞不稳定,有时难以和其他细胞进行严格区别。

Most of these cells display scattered growth, are generally not fragmented. This type of cell is unstable and sometimes difficult to distinguish from other cell types.

4. 多形性细胞型 Polymorphic cell type

难以确定其稳定形态的细胞,常归于此类,如神经细胞等。

Cells with unstable or diverse morphologies, including nerve cells, are often placed in this category.

(二)悬浮型 Suspension-dependent type

有一些类型的细胞在体外培养时不需要贴附,而是悬浮生长。这些细胞的胞体常呈圆形,多见于一些造血系肿瘤细胞,其特点是悬浮型细胞生长速度较快、传代方便。常见的U937、HL60、K562造血系肿瘤细胞均属此种类型。

Some types of cells grow in suspension rather than attachment *in vitro*. The cell bodies of these cells are usually round, such as those observed for hematopoietic tumor cells. The characteristics of these cells include fast growth rates and convenient passage. U937, HL60 and K562 hematopoietic tumor cells belong to this type.

二、体外培养细胞与体内细胞的差异 Differences between cultured cells *in vitro* and *in vivo*

细胞离体后,失去了神经体液的调节和细胞间相互作用的影响,生活在缺乏动态平衡的相对稳定环境中。体外培养的正常细胞成为一种在特定条件下生长的细胞群体。它们既保持着与体内细胞相同的基本结构和功能,也出现了一些不同于机体细胞的性状,主要表现在:①失去原有组织结构和细胞形态,如体外培养的肌肉细胞表现出纤维化的特点;②分化减弱或不显,出现类似"返祖"现象(去分化),细胞的形态功能趋向单一化,或生存一定时间后衰退死亡;③发生转化获得永生,变成可无限生长的系或恶性细胞系,或变成具有恶性性状的细胞群。

After the cells are isolated, they lose the regulation by secreted growth factors and direct intercellular interactions, living in a relatively stable environment, but lacking dynamic balance. Normal cells cultured *in vitro* become a colony of cells growing under specific conditions. They often retain the same basic structure and functions as cells *in vivo*, but may also display properties different from those cells. These differences include: ①Loss of original tissue structure and cell morphology, for example, muscle cells cultured *in vitro* may exhibit fibrotic characteristics. ②Differentiation characteristics may weaken and become less apparent, and morphologies and functions of cells become more uniform or decline. Cells may also die after a certain period of survival. ③The transformed cells acquire immortality, permitting indefinite growth in culture, and in some cases develop malignant characteristics.

三、培养细胞的生长特点　Growth characteristics of subcultured cells *in vitro*

（一）贴附　Attach

大多数哺乳动物细胞在体外生长时需附着在一定底物如塑料、胶原、玻璃或其他细胞做成的饲养层细胞上才能生长、分裂。贴附之前的细胞一般为球体样，在一些特殊的能促进细胞贴附的物质如Ⅲ型胶原、血清扩展因子的帮助下，细胞先吸附到底物上，随后与底物附着并伸展成一定的形状。

Most mammalian cells grow and divide *in vitro* by attaching to specific substrates such as plastics，collagen，glass or feeding layer cells. Before attachment，cells are usually spherical. Cells attach to substrates and then stretch to attain certain shapes with the help of molecules that promote adhesion，such as type Ⅲ collagen serum extension factors.

不同细胞的贴附能力不同，如巨噬细胞、成纤维细胞等的贴附能力较强，能在数分钟至数十分钟内贴附到固相表面；而神经元、羊水细胞等的贴附能力则较弱，一般需要数小时乃至更长的时间才能贴附到固相表面。

Different cells have different attachment abilities. For example，macrophagocytes and fibroblasts develop strong attachments to solid surfaces within several minutes. By contrast，neurons and amniotic fluid cells develop weak attachments to solid surfaces，which often take several hours or even longer to develop.

（二）接触抑制与密度依赖性　Contact inhibition and density dependence

对于相当一部分体外培养的贴附依赖型细胞来说，随着细胞不断地生长与分裂，当相邻两个细胞彼此靠近时，其中之一或两个细胞便会停止移动而不至于重叠起来，转而朝向未有细胞生长的空间，这种现象被称为接触抑制（contact inhibition）。而进一步的生长会使细胞密度变得越来越大直至形成一个细胞单层。在此过程中，细胞与培养基接触的面积也会相应减少。此时，细胞的分裂便会停止，但细胞还会存活一段时间，这种现象被称为密度抑制（density inhibition）或密度依赖性（density dependence）。通常，细胞的这种密度依赖性与培养基中血清的浓度关系密切。

For many types of adherent cells cultured *in vitro*，cells that contact other cells will stop moving and turn toward an unoccupied the space on the surface they are growing on. This phenomenon is called contact inhibition. Further growth will increase cell density until a contiguous，single cell layer is formed. By this process，the area of contact between cells and culture medium is reduced. At this time，cell division will stop，but cells will continue to survive，at least temporally，a phenomenon termed density inhibition or density dependence. Density dependence of cells is often closely related to the concentration of serum in the medium.

与体外培养的正常细胞不同，转化细胞或恶变的肿瘤细胞的接触抑制特性降低或丧失，导致细胞重叠生长。同时，转化细胞或恶变的肿瘤细胞的密度依赖性调节也常常降低，对血清的依赖性也降低，可以生长到一个较高的终末细胞密度。

Unlike normal cells cultured *in vitro*，contact inhibition of transformed cells or malignant tumor cells is reduced or lost, resulting in an overlapping pattern of cell growth. Density-dependent regulation and dependence on serum is also reduced for transformed cells and malignant tumor cells, resulting in cultures that reach higher terminal cell densities.

四、体外培养细胞的生长过程　Growth process of cultured cells *in vitro*

体外生长的培养细胞受营养条件、生长空间等因素的限制,当细胞增殖达到一定密度后,需要分离出一部分细胞和更新营养液进行扩大培养,此过程称传代(subculture)。每次传代以后,细胞的生长和增殖过程都会受一定的影响。加之很多细胞特别是正常细胞,其在体外的生存也不是无限的过程,这就使得细胞在体外培养时的生长过程与体内有着一系列的不同。

In vitro growth of cultured cells is limited by nutrient conditions, growth space and other factors. When cells proliferate to a certain density, it is necessary to isolate some cells and resupply nutrients for expanded culture. This process is called subculture or passage. After each passage, the growth and proliferation of cells will be affected. In addition, many cells, especially normal cells, which cannot survive indefinitely *in vitro*, may develop altered characteristics as they grow in culture compared to growth *in vivo*.

（一）培养细胞的生命期　Life span of cultured cells

培养细胞的生命期是细胞在培养过程中持续增殖和生长的时间。体内组织细胞的生存期与完整机体的死亡衰老基本一致。体外培养细胞的生命期与细胞的种类、性状和原供体的年龄等情况密切相关。比如,来源自人胚的二倍体成纤维细胞可在体外连续传代 30～50 代,150～300 个细胞增殖周期,相当于一年左右的生存时间。相比之下,那些来自成体或衰老个体的细胞生存时间则较短,如体外培养的肝细胞或肾细胞一般仅能传几代或十几代。

通常,体外培养细胞的生命期大致可分为原代培养期、传代期、衰退期 3 个阶段。

The life span of culture cells is defined as the time of continuous proliferation and growth in culture. The survival time of tissue cells *in vivo* is basically the same as that of the whole organism. The life span of cultured cells *in vitro* is closely related to the type, character and age of their source. For example, diploid fibroblasts derived from human embryos can be subcultured continuously for 30 to 50 passages or a total of 150 to 300 cells divisions. In contrast, cells derived from adult or senile individuals generally survive for shorter periods of time. Hepatocytes or kidney cells, for example, can only passaged for several generations.

Generally, the life span of cultured cells *in vitro* can be roughly divided into three stages: primary culture period, passage period and recession period.

1. 原代培养期　Primary culture period

原代培养也称初代培养,是从机体中取出细胞接种培养到第一次传代之前的阶段。此期的细胞呈现出活跃移动的特点,可见细胞分裂,但不旺盛。处于原代培养阶段的细胞与体内原组织在形态、结构和功能活动上有很大的相似性。细胞群具有明显的异质性,细胞间的相互依存性强,在软琼脂培养基培养时细胞集落形成率很低。

Primary culture, also known as first generation culture, is the stage during which cells are removed from the body and cultured to the first passage. The cells during this phase are characterized by active movement, showing cell division, but are not strong. The cells during the primary culture stage share many similarities with the original tissues with respect to morphological structures and functional activities. Cell populations have obvious heterogeneity and strong interdependence and rates of colony formation are very low for cells cultured on a soft agar medium.

2. 传代期 Passage period

传代期通常是培养细胞生命期中持续时间最长的时期,原代培养的细胞经传代后常被称做细胞系(cell line)。一般情况下,正常体细胞在传代 10～50 次后,细胞的分裂能力就会逐渐减弱,甚至完全丧失,细胞便进入衰退期。

The passage period is usually the longest period in the life of cultured cells. Primary cultured cells are often called "cell lines" after passage. Normally, after 10 to 50 passages of normal somatic cells, the ability of cell division will gradually weaken, or even be completely lost, after which the cells will enter a recession period.

3. 衰退期 Recession period

处于衰退期的培养细胞,增殖速率已经变得很慢或不再增殖,直至最后衰退死亡。

The proliferation rates of cultured cells during the recession stage become very slow or fall to zero until the final recession and death.

以上主要是针对体外培养的机体正常细胞,对于体外发生转化的细胞和肿瘤细胞而言,永生性(immortality)或恶型性(malignancy)的获得使得这类细胞具有持久的增殖能力,这样的细胞群体常被称为无限细胞系(infinite cell line)或连续细胞系(continuous cell line)。

The above periods chiefly apply to normal (non-transformed) cells cultured *in vitro*. For transformed cells and cancer cells, the acquisition of immortality or malignancy allows these cells to proliferate indefinitely in cell culture. Populations of these cells are often referred to as infinite cell lines or continuous cell lines.

（二）培养细胞的一代生存期 Generation survival period of cultured cells

所谓培养细胞的"一代生存期"是指从细胞接种后到再次传代培养之前的这一段时间,与细胞世代(generation)或倍增(doubling)时间不同。例如,某一细胞系为第 60 代细胞,即指该细胞系已传代了 60 次。就培养细胞的一代生存期而言,细胞通常可以倍增 3～6 次。

培养细胞的一代生存期,一般可被分为潜伏期、对数生长期和停滞期 3 个阶段。

The length of one generation of cultured cells is the period from the time of cell inoculation to the time before passage (subculture), which is different from the cell division or doubling time. For example, a cell line is its 60th generation means that the cell line has been passaged 60 times. During one generation survival time, cells can typically undergo cell division 3 to 6 times.

One generation of cultured cells can be divided into three stages: latent phase, exponential phase and stationary phase.

1. 潜伏期 Latent phase

以贴附生长的培养细胞为例,刚刚经历传代接种的细胞,常在培养基中呈现悬浮状态,此时细胞的胞质回缩,胞体呈圆球形。紧接着,悬浮细胞便会贴附于底物表面上,此过程称为贴壁。各种细胞贴附速度并不相同,这与培养细胞的种类、培养基成分和底物的理化性质等密切相关。待细胞贴附于支持物后,细胞便开始进一步伸展成极性细胞,但这距离细胞进入生长和增殖期还有一定时间,称为潜伏期(latent phase)。细胞潜伏期的长短与细胞接种密度、细胞种类以及培养基性质等密切相关。通常,原代培养细胞的潜伏期较长,需24~96 h或更长时间;而连续细胞系细胞的潜伏期则较短,仅6~24 h。细胞接种密度大时潜伏期常会变短。

For example，adherent cells that have just been subcultured often remain suspended in culture medium for varying lengths of time. During this phase，cellular cytoplasm retracts and cell bodies become round. The suspended cells eventually attach to the surface of the substrate，a process known as adherence. The rate of attachment varies among different types of cells and is also influenced by the composition of culture medium and the physical and chemical properties of substrates. After the cells attach to the supporting substrate，their morphologies become elongated，but a variable lag occurs before the cells enter the growth and proliferation phase. This period is called the latent phase. The length of the latent phase varies with the cell inoculation density，cell type and the nature of culture medium. Generally，the latent phase of primary cultured cells is about 24 to 96 hours or longer，while that of continuous cell lines is only 6 to 24 hours. In addition，the latent phase is often shortened when the cell inoculation density is high.

2. 对数生长期 Exponential phase

当细胞分裂象开始出现并逐渐增多,便标志着潜伏期的结束和对数生长期的开始。对数生长期是细胞增殖分裂最旺盛的阶段。对数生长期细胞分裂象数量的多少常作为判定细胞生长旺盛与否的重要标志,一般用分裂指数(mitotic index,MI)来表示。分裂指数是指分裂象在整个细胞群中所占的百分比。体外培养细胞的分裂指数受细胞种类、培养液成分、营养条件、pH值、培养温度等多种因素影响。一般细胞的分裂指数多介于0.1%~0.5%,原代细胞分裂指数较低,连续细胞分裂指数可高达3%~5%。对数生长期是细胞一代生存期中活力最好的时期,是进行各种实验最好和最主要的阶段。

The appearance and gradual increase in cell division marks the end of the latent phase and the beginning of the exponential phase. exponential phase is the most vigorous stage of cell proliferation and division. The number of mitotic cells in exponential phase is often used as to quantify cell growth. The percentage of mitotic cells in the cell population is termed the mitotic index（MI）. The mitotic index of cultured cells is influenced by many factors，including as cell type，culture medium composition，nutritional conditions，pH，and incubator temperature. In general，the mitotic index of cells ranges from 0.1% to 0.5%. The mitotic index of primary cells is low. The mitotic index of continuous cells can reach as high as 3% to 5%. Exponential phase is the most vigorous period in the survival period of cell generation, and the best and most important stage for many experiments.

3. 停滞期　Stationary phase

当细胞数量达饱和密度后，细胞停止增殖，进入停滞期。此时细胞数量不再增加，故也称平台期（plateau phase）。处于此期的细胞虽不增殖，但仍有代谢活动；而随着培养液中营养渐趋耗尽，代谢产物的积累、pH 值的降低，此时需要进行及时的传代培养，否则细胞会因营养匮乏、中毒等原因，发生形态改变，甚至从底物脱落死亡。

When cultured cells reach saturated density, cell division ceases and the cells enter a stationary phase. During this phase, the number of cells does not increase, so it is also referred to as a plateau phase. Although cells in this stage do not proliferate, they are still metabolically active. However, with the gradual depletion of nutrients in the culture medium, the accumulation of metabolites and the decrease in medium pH, timely subculture is required. Cells in stagnated cultures undergo morphological changes due to lack of nutrients and poisoning by toxic metabolic substrates and eventually detach from culture substrate and die.

第三节 ◎ 原代培养与传代培养
Primary culture and subculture

一、原代培养　Primary culture

将动物机体中待培养组织取出，然后通过各种消化性酶（如胰蛋白酶）消化，或用机械方法处理，将组织分离成单细胞，最后添加适当的培养基培养，使细胞得以生存、生长和繁殖的过程称为原代培养。原代培养的细胞与机体细胞在形态、结构、功能等方面非常接近，是药理等实验重要的研究材料。本节以新生小鼠肝细胞的原代培养为例。

The process of extracting tissue from animal bodies and digesting it with various digestive enzymes (such as trypsin) or mechanical treatment, separating the tissue into single cells, and finally adding appropriate medium to culture, so that cells can survive, grow and reproduce is called primary culture. Primary cultured cells are very similar to cells within the original tissues with respect to morphology, structure and function, and are often used as research materials in pharmacological experiments.

（一）仪器与试剂　Required equipment and reagents

超净工作台、细胞培养箱、离心机、倒置显微镜、普通光学显微镜、离心管、培养瓶、平皿、移液管、血细胞计数板、水浴锅、0.25% 的胰蛋白酶液（含 0.02% EDTA）、RPMI 1640 细胞培养基（含 20% 的 FBS）、Hank's 平衡盐溶液（Hank's balanced salt solution，HBSS）、75% 乙醇、碘酒。

Laminar flow cabinet, cell culture incubator, centrifuge, inverted microscope, bright-field microscope, centrifuge tubes, culture flasks, plates, pipettes, hemocytometer, water bath, 0. 25% trypsin (0. 02% EDTA solution), RPMI 1640 medium (20% FBS), Hank's balanced salt solution (HBSS), 75% ethanol solution, iodine.

（二）操作步骤 **Protocols**

1. 胰蛋白酶消化法 Trypsin digestion method

（1）将新生小鼠颈椎脱臼处死,置 75%乙醇泡 2～3 s,再用碘酒消毒腹部,用纱布将小鼠包裹后带入超净台内,解剖取肝脏,放入一玻璃平皿中。

Pull the cervical spine of neonatal mice to induce death, soak the body in 75% ethanol solution for 2 to 3 seconds, sterilize the abdomen with iodine, wrap the body with gauze, place it in the laminar flow cabinet, dissect and remove the liver and put it on to a glass plate.

（2）用 HBSS 洗涤 3 次,并剔除脂肪、结缔组织和血液等杂物,然后用手术剪将肝脏剪成 1 mm×1 mm×1 mm 大小的组织块,再用 HBSS 洗涤 3 次。

Wash the liver three times with HBSS, and remove the fat, connective tissue, blood and other debris. Cut the liver into 1 mm×1 mm×1 mm size tissue blocks with a surgical scissors and wash these three times with HBSS.

（3）将组织块转移至一离心管中,视组织块的多少加入 5～6 倍体积的 0.25%胰蛋白酶液(37℃预温)。

Transfer the tissue blocks into a centrifuge tube and containing 0. 25% trypsin digestion solution preheated at 37℃ at 5 to 6 times the volume of the tissue blocks.

（4）待大部分细胞被消化成为单细胞后,加入 3～5 ml RPMI 1640 细胞培养基及时终止胰蛋白酶的消化作用。

After most of the cells have separated into single cells, terminate trypsin digestion by addition of 3 to 5 ml RPMI 1640 medium.

（5）将上述细胞悬液转移至一离心管中,1 000 r/min,离心 5 min,弃上清液。

Transfer the cell suspension to a centrifugal tube, centrifuge at 1 000 r/min for 5 min, and discard the supernatant.

（6）加入 HBSS 5 ml,重悬细胞,然后 1 000 r/min,离心 5 min,弃上清液。

Add 5 ml of HBSS, resuspend the cells, and repeat the previous step.

（7）加入 1～2 ml 培养基重悬细胞,血细胞计数板计数细胞密度。

Resuspend the cells in 1 to 2 ml of the culture medium, and measure cell density using a hemocytometer.

（8）在细胞计数的基础之上,利用培养基将细胞密度调整到 5×10^5 个/ml 左右,然后将细胞悬液转移(分装)至相应大小的细胞培养瓶中,置细胞培养箱中 37℃培养。

On the basis of the cell count, adjust the cell density to about 5×10^5 cells/ml with culture medium, transfer the cell suspension to an appropriately sized cell culture flask, and incubate at 37℃ in the cell culture incubator.

2. 组织块法 Tissue block method

（1）第一步、第二步与胰蛋白酶消化法相同。

Steps 1 and 2 are the same as for the trypsin digestion method.

（2）将用 HBSS 洗涤后的组织块直接转移到培养瓶，贴附在培养瓶的底面（凹面，生长面）。

Transfer tissue blocks washed with HBSS directly to a culture flask and attach the bottom of the culture flask（concave surface，growth surface）.

（3）将培养瓶翻转，使培养瓶的生长面朝上，然后加入适量培养基至瓶中，应避免培养液与组织块接触。

Turn the culture flask upside down so that the growth side of the culture flask is facing up，and then add the appropriate amount of culture medium to the bottle，avoiding contact between the culture solution and the tissue blocks.

（4）将培养瓶小心转移至细胞培养箱中，37℃静置 2～3 h，然后轻轻翻转培养瓶，使培养瓶生长面的组织浸入培养基中（勿使组织漂起），继续培养。

Carefully transfer the culture flask to a cell culture incubator set at 37℃ for 2 to 3 hours，then gently invert the culture flask，so that the growth surface tissue of the culture flask is immersed in the culture medium（do not let the tissue float）and continue to culture.

（三）注意事项 Notes

（1）自取材开始，保持所有组织细胞处于无菌环境。细胞计数可在有菌环境中进行。

From the beginning of sampling，maintain all tissues and cells under aseptic conditions；cell counts can be performed in any environment.

（2）75%乙醇浸泡消毒的时间不宜过长，以免乙醇从口和肛门浸入小鼠体内。

The time of disinfection in 75% ethanol solution should be short，so as not to allow infiltration of ethanol to the mice from the mouth and anus.

（3）等组织块周围长出单细胞层后将组织块剔除，便可收获细胞或进行传代培养。

After the monolayer grows around the tissue block and the tissue block has been removed，the cells can be harvested or subcultured.

（4）胰蛋白酶消化的时间长短与组织细胞的幼嫩程度、数量以及酶的活力等因素密切相关。此外，在消化过程中应密切观察，及时吹打，避免消化过度。

The time of trypsin digestion is closely related to the freshness，quantity of tissue cells and enzyme activity. In addition，close observation should be made in the digestion process to prevent excessive digestion.

二、细胞传代培养 Cell subculture

当细胞在培养瓶长成致密的单层后，通常已经没有足够的生长空间和营养条件满足细胞进一步生长的需求。为使细胞能继续生长，并使细胞的数量扩大，就必须进行传代再培养。同时，传代培养也是保存细胞的方法，是利用培养细胞进行各种实验的必经过程。通常，悬浮型细胞可通过直接补充培养基后再分瓶的方法进行传代，方法相对简单，而贴附型细胞则需要消化后才能分瓶培养。

When cells have grown into a dense monolayer in culture flasks, there is usually insufficient growth space and nutrient conditions to support further cell growth. To enable cells to continue to grow and expand in number, it is necessary to subculture and re-culture. Subculture is also a way to preserve cells and required for various experiments. Suspension cell cultures can be subcultured by simply adding culture medium and distributing the cultures one or more new culture flasks. By contrast, adherent cells need to be gently digested before being cultured in separate bottles.

（一）仪器与试剂　Required equipment and reagents

超净工作台、细胞培养箱、离心机、离心管、倒置显微镜、吸管、废液缸、培养瓶、移液管、0.25%的胰蛋白酶液（含0.02%EDTA）、DMEM细胞培养基（含10%FBS）、HBSS。

Laminar flow cabinet, cell incubator, centrifuge, centrifuge tube, inverted microscope, pipette, waste tank, culture flask, pipette, 0.25% trypsin/0.02% EDTA solution, DMEM medium（20% FBS）, HBSS.

（二）操作步骤　Protocols

1. 贴附依赖型细胞的传代培养　Subculture of adherent cells

（1）弃去培养瓶中的培养液。

Discard the original culture medium in culture flask, without disturbing the attached cells.

（2）加入1～2 ml 0.25%胰蛋白酶液，使所有细胞都能浸入溶液中，室温或37℃消化。

Add 1 to 2 ml of 0.25% trypsin solution so that all cells are covered by the solution and incubate at room temperature or 37℃.

（3）利用倒置显微镜或肉眼观察细胞的消化状况。随着时间的推移，原本贴壁的细胞会逐渐变圆，并开始脱落。

Observe the state of the cells using an inverted microscope or by eye. Over time, the adherent cells will gradually become round and begin to detach from the surface of the culture flask.

（4）待到消化充分后，及时加入10 ml HBSS终止消化。

After digestion, terminate the process by adding 10 ml of HBSS.

（5）用吸管将贴壁的细胞吹打成悬液，转移至离心管中，1 000 r/min，离心5 min，弃上清液。

Gently dislodge the remaining adherent cells by repeated pipetting and transfer the suspended cells into a centrifuge tube. Centrifuge at 1 000 r/min for 5 min and discard the supernatant.

（6）用10～15 ml DMEM细胞培养基重悬细胞，并将其分装到2～3个培养瓶中，37℃下继续培养。

Resuspend the cells in 10 to 15 ml of fresh DMEM medium, and dispense them into two to three flasks, and continue to culture at 37℃.

(7) 过夜观察细胞的贴壁及生长状况。

Carefully observe the degree of cell attachment and growth after overnight incubation.

2. 悬浮型细胞的传代培养　Subculture of suspension cells

悬浮型细胞的传代培养要比贴附依赖型细胞简单得多,通常有两种方法。

Subculture of suspension cells is much simpler than subculture of adherent cells, and one of two methods is often used.

(1) 直接给待传代的培养瓶中补充一定量的新鲜培养基,然后进行分装。

Add an appropriate amount of fresh medium directly to the culture flask containing cells to be passaged and dispense into fresh culture flasks.

(2) 先通过离心弃掉营养匮乏的旧培养基,再用适量的新鲜培养基重悬细胞沉淀物,最后将其分装至培养瓶中。

Centrifuge the culture medium containing the suspended cells and discard the supernatant. Resuspend the cellular pellet with an appropriate amount of fresh medium, dispense it into the fresh culture flasks.

(三) 注意事项　Notes

(1) 传代的比例取决于细胞的生长状态、生长速度以及实验的目的要求等因素,通常按照 1∶2 或 1∶3 的比例进行传代。

The fold ratio of each passage depends on factors such as cell growth status, growth rate and the experimental goals. Passage ratios of 1∶2 or 1∶3 are often used.

(2) 传代培养时,消化液的作用时间受到诸多因素的影响,消化过程应密切观察细胞的形态变化,避免消化过度。

The appropriate duration of trypsin digestion used for passaging adherent cells is influenced by many factors. For this reason, changes in cellular morphology should be closely observed to avoid over-digestion.

(3) 首次传代的细胞可适当增加其接种量,以促进其生存与增殖。

Cells that are passaged for the first time should be passaged at low fold ratios to promote survival and proliferation.

三、附录　Appendix

(一) 胰蛋白酶液的配制　Trypsin solution

精确称取 0.25 g 胰蛋白酶(活力为 1∶250),加入 100 ml 不含 Ca^{2+}、Mg^{2+} 的 HBSS 中溶解,滤器过滤除菌,4℃保存。胰蛋白酶溶液中也可加入 EDTA,其终浓度为 0.02%。

Accurately weigh 0.25 g of trypsin (1∶250 viability), dissolve in 100 ml of Ca^{2+} and Mg^{2+}-free HBSS, filter sterilize and store at 4℃. EDTA can also be added to the trypsin solution at a final concentration of 0.02%.

(二) Hank's 平衡盐溶液的配制　Hank's balanced salt solution(HBSS)

KH_2PO_4 0.06 g, NaCl 8.0 g, $NaHCO_3$ 0.35 g, KCl 0.4 g, 葡萄糖 1.0 g, Na_2HPO_4 •

H₂O 0.06 g，酚红 0.02 g，加超纯水至 1 000 ml，过滤除菌或高压灭菌，分装后 4℃ 保存。

KH₂PO₄ 0.06 g，NaCl 8.0 g，NaHCO₃ 0.35 g，KCl 0.4 g，glucose 1.0 g，Na₂HPO₄ · H₂O 0.06 g and phenol red 0.02 g in 1 000 ml ultrapure water，filter sterilize or autoclave，and store at 4℃ after dispensing.

（三）RPMI 1640 培养基的制备与消毒　RPMI 1640 medium

先将培养基粉剂加入培养液体积 2/3 的超纯水中，并用超纯水冲洗包装袋 2～3 次（冲洗液一并加入培养基中），充分搅拌至粉剂全部溶解，并按照包装说明书添加一定的药品。然后用注射器向培养基中加入配制好的青霉素、链霉素液各 0.5 ml，使青霉素、链霉素的浓度最终各为 100 U/ml。然后用盐酸和 NaOH 调 pH 到 7.2 左右。最后定容至 1 000 ml，摇匀。配制好的培养基通常用滤器过滤除菌，将过滤好的培养液分装入小瓶内置于 4℃ 冰箱内待用。

Add pre-formulated RPMI 1640 medium powder to 2/3 final culture medium volume ultrapure water. Rinse the bag that contained the medium powder 2 to 3 times with ultrapure water，adding each rinse to the culture medium. Stir well until the powder is completely dissolved，following the manufacturer's instructions. Add premade 0.5 ml streptomycin and penicillin solution using a syringe to a final streptomycin and penicillin concentration of 100 U/ml. Adjust the pH of the medium about 7.2 with hydrochloric acid and NaOH. Finally，add ultrapure water to a final volume of 1 000 ml and shake well. The culture medium is usually filtered and then filter-sterilized. Aliquots of the sterilized culture medium can be stored at 4℃ for future use.

第四节 ⊙ 细胞系的建立
Establishment of cell lines

原代培养的细胞经第一次传代培养后常被称为"细胞系"（cell line）。由某一细胞系分离出来、在性状上与原细胞系有一定差异的细胞系，常被称为该细胞系的"亚系"（subline）。从一个经过鉴定的细胞系采用选择法或单细胞克隆进一步所得到的细胞群，常被称"细胞株"（cell strain）。由原细胞株进一步分离培养出的与原株性状不同的细胞群，又被称为"亚株"（substrain）。

Primary cultured cells are often called a cell "line" after their first subculture. Cell lines isolated from a previously prepared cell line that differ in traits from the original cell line are often referred to as "sublines" of the original cell line. A population of cells obtained by selection or single cell cloning from an identified cell line is often referred to as a "cell strain." A cell population derived from an original cell strain，but displaying different properties is often called a cell "substrain".

一、细胞系的建立　Establishment of cell lines

细胞建系的一般程序包括原代培养、第一次传代、常规传代、冻存与复苏等过程。所涉及的原代培养、第一次传代、常规传代、冻存与复苏等过程的具体方法与相关的常规细胞培养技术相同。

The general procedure for establishing a new cell line includes primary culture，first passage，routine passage，freezing and thawing. The specific methods involved in these processes are the same as those for conventional primary culture.

用于建系的细胞通常有一些特别的要求。应详细说明细胞供体所属物种、供体的年龄、性别、取材的器官或组织。如系肿瘤组织，还应说明临床病理诊断结果，组织来源以及病例号等。各种细胞都有自己比较适应的生存环境，因此应指明适合该细胞系生长的培养基、血清种类、浓度以及细胞生存的适宜 pH 值等。

The cells used to establish a cell line usually have specific requirements. Information concerning the source of new cell lines，including species，age，sex，and organs or tissue taken should be specified in detail. For tumor tissue，clinicopathological diagnosis，tissue origin and case number should also be recorded. Different types of cells have their own requirements for *in vitro* culture，so the optimal medium type，serum type and concentration，and pH required for cell survival should be indicated.

二、细胞系的鉴定、管理　Authentication and management of cell lines

(一)细胞系的鉴定　Authentication of cell lines

要求能提供细胞一般和特殊的生物学性状指标，包括：细胞的一般形态、特异性结构、细胞生长曲线、分裂指数、倍增时间、接种率、染色体分析、同工酶检查和 DNA 指纹图谱等。

Authentication of cell lines requires information about the general and specific biological characteristics of the cells. General and specific cellular characteristics include：cell morphology，cell growth curve and division index，doubling time，results of chromosome，isozyme，and DNA fingerprinting analyses.

1. 对正常细胞系的鉴定　Authentication of normal cell lines

对正常细胞系的鉴定主要围绕以下 4 个方面进行：①鉴定细胞的种系来源，常用方法主要有染色体分析、同工酶分析、DNA 指纹图谱等技术；②鉴定细胞的组织来源，可通过形态学检测、组织特异性抗原检测等进行鉴定；③细胞是否发生转化和恶变，主要通过核型分析、细胞生长行为观察(是否丧失接触抑制)、裸鼠成瘤实验等进行鉴定；④细胞有无发生交叉污染，主要通过同工酶及 DNA 指纹图谱技术进行鉴定。

Authentication of normal cell lines mainly concerns the following four aspects：①Identification of germline sources of cells using methods such as chromosome analysis，isozyme analysis，and DNA fingerprinting；②The tissue source of cells can be identified by morphology，and tissue-specific antigens；③Whether the cells have undergone transformation or malignancy is mainly determined by karyotype analysis，observation of cell growth behavior（for example，loss of contact inhibition），and tumorigenesis experiments using nude mice；④Cross-contamination of cells can detected by isozyme and/or DNA fingerprinting analyses.

2. 对肿瘤细胞系的鉴定　Authentication of tumor cell lines

对肿瘤细胞系的鉴定主要围绕其恶型性展开,染色体的异常、接触抑制和密度依赖生长特性的改变、集落形成能力、裸鼠成瘤、动物体内的侵袭生长,以及某些基因、分子水平的特征均是肿瘤细胞鉴定的方向。

The identification of tumor cell lines mainly focuses on their malignancy, abnormal chromosomes, contact inhibition and density-dependent growth characteristics, colony forming ability, tumor formation in nude mice, invasion and growth in animals, and expression of specific gene and molecules. The trend is for molecular level characterization of tumor cells.

(二) 细胞系的管理 Management of cell lines

对已建立和经过鉴定的细胞系,一般除保留在建立者的实验室外,为了科研交流的方便和细胞系的稳定性,国际上通行的惯例是将其保存在细胞库中。在国际上,美、英和日本等国已建有细胞库。其中,美国的 ATCC(american type culture collecion)作为美国国立癌症研究所(NCI)和美国卫生研究所(NIH)的细胞资源库,也是世界卫生组织(WHO)的国际细胞培养中心。ATCC 是世界上最大的细胞库,现存细胞系超过数千种。ATCC 接纳来自世界各国已经鉴定的细胞予以储存,同时也向世界各国的研究者或实验室提供研究用细胞。除美国的 ATCC(网址:http://www.atcc.org)之外,欧洲细胞培养物收藏中心(ECACC)也是重要的细胞库,建立于 1984 年,其网址为:http://www.ecacc.org.uk/。

Established and identified cell lines are generally stored in the laboratories of the founders. For the convenience of scientific research and communication and the stability of the cell lines, it is also a common international practice to store cell lines in the cell banks. Cell banks have been established in the United States, Britain and Japan. Among these, the American ATCC (American type culture collection), as the cell resource bank of the National Cancer Institute (NCI) and the National Institutes of Health (NIH), is the International Culture Cell Documentation Center of the World Health Organization (WHO). ATCC accepts for storage identified cell lines from all over the world, and also provides cells to researchers and laboratories around the world. In addition to ATCC (website: http://www.atcc.org) in the United States, the European Cell Culture Collection Centre (ECACC) is also an important cell bank established in 1984. Its website is http://www.ecacc.org.uk/.

此外,对于已建立的各种细胞系或细胞株习惯上都给予名称。细胞的命名无严格统一规定,大多采用有一定意义缩写字或代号表示。例如,HeLa 为供体患者的姓名缩写;中国地鼠卵巢细胞(Chinese hamster ovary,CHO),为英文单词的首位字母组成;宫-743 意为1974 年 3 月建立的宫颈癌上皮细胞;NIH3T3 是因 NIH 建立,每 3 天传代,每次接种 3×10^5 个细胞/毫升而得名。

It is customary to give names to established cell lines or cell strains. There are no strict or uniform rules for cell nomenclature, most of which are expressed by abbreviations or codes with certain meanings. For example: HeLa: abbreviation for the name of the donor patient (Helen Lane); CHO: Chinese hamster ovary, based on the first letter of each English word；Gong-743：meaning cervical cancer epithelial cells established in March 1974；NIH3T3：established by the National Institutes of Health (NIH) and passaged every three days, each time by inoculating 3×10^5 cells/ml.

第五节 ◎ 细胞的冻存与复苏
Freezing and thawing of cells

为了保存细胞,特别是不易获得的突变型细胞或细胞株,要将细胞冻存。通常使用－196℃的液氮进行细胞冻存,冻存过程中需要缓慢冷冻。因为细胞在不加任何保护剂的情况下直接冻存,细胞内外的水分会很快形成冰晶,并且随冰晶数量增多,会导致细胞脱水及渗透压增高等后果,从而造成细胞的损伤。目前,细胞冻存多采用甘油或二甲基亚砜作为保护剂。这两种物质在低温冷冻后对细胞均无明显毒性,并且分子量小,溶解度大,易穿透细胞,可使冰点下降,提高细胞膜对水的通透性;加上缓慢冻存可使细胞内的水分渗出细胞外,在胞外形成冰晶,减少细胞内冰晶的形成,从而减少冰晶对细胞的损伤。

复苏细胞与冻存的要求相反,应采用快速融化的手段。这样可保证细胞外冰晶在很短的时间内融化,并避免由于缓慢融化使水分渗入细胞内形成胞内再结晶对细胞造成损害。

To preserve cells，especially mutant cells or cell lines that are not readily available，cells should be cryopreserved. The temperature of cryopreservation is generally － 196℃ with liquid nitrogen. Cells should be slowly frozen when they are cryopreserved. Because the cells freeze directly without any protective agent，the water inside and outside the cells will quickly form ice crystals，and as the number of ice crystals increases，it will lead to cell dehydration and increase osmotic pressure，resulting in cell damage. At present，glycerol or dimethyl sulfoxide is used as a protective agent for cell cryopreservation. These two substances have no obvious toxicity to cells after freezing at a low temperature，and have small molecular weight，large solubility，easy to penetrate cells，which can decrease the freezing point and improve the water permeability of cell membranes. In addition，slow cryopreservation can make the water in cells seep out of cells，form ice crystals in the cell surface and reduce the formation of ice crystals inside the cells，thereby reducing cell damage caused by ice crystal formation.

By contrast to slow cryopreservation，resuscitation or cells should include rapid thawing. This ensures that extracellular ice crystals rapidly melt，thereby avoiding damage to the cells caused by the infiltration of water that can occur when cells are thawed slowly.

一、细胞的冻存　Freezing of cells

（一）仪器与试剂　Required equipment and reagents

细胞培养箱、超净台、液氮罐、普通冰箱、－80℃超低温冰箱、离心机、冻存管、离心管、冻存盒、倒置显微镜、吸管、废液缸、0.25%的胰蛋白酶液(含0.02%EDTA)、细胞冻存液[10 ml

体系：含 7 ml 培养基、2 ml FBS、1 ml 甘油或二甲基亚砜(dimethyl sulfoxide，DMSO)]、细胞培养基(如添加有 10%FBS 的 RPMI 1640)等。

Cell culture incubator，laminar flow cabinet，liquid nitrogen tank，general refrigerator，－80℃ ultra-low temperature refrigerator，centrifuge，cryogenic tube，centrifuge tube，freezing container inverted microscope，pipette，waste tank，0.25% trypsin(0.02% EDTA) solution，cell cryopreservation solution (10 ml system：containing 7 ml medium，2 ml FBS，1 ml glycerol or DMSO)，cell culture medium (such as RPMI 1640 with 10% FBS added).

（二）操作步骤 Protocols

（1）取旺盛生长的、已基本上快要长满细胞的培养瓶，在超净台内小心吸干瓶内培养液。给每个培养瓶中加入 1～2 ml 胰蛋白酶液，37℃ 消化细胞。

Take a vigorously growing culture flask that is almost full of cells and carefully remove the culture medium. Add 1 to 2 ml of trypsin solution to each culture flask，and incubate at 37℃.

（2）待大部分细胞从瓶壁脱落下来后，加入 3～5 ml 细胞培养基终止消化。

After most of the cells become detached from the flask inner surface，add 3 to 5 ml of cell culture medium terminate the digestion.

（3）700～800 r/min 离心 5 min，收集细胞沉淀物。

Centrifuge at 700 to 800 r/min （about $200 \times g$） for 5 min and remove the supernatant.

（4）加入适量细胞冻存液，调整细胞密度在$(1～10) \times 10^6$ 个/ml。

Resuspend the cellular pellet in an appropriate volume of cell cryopreservation solution，adjusting the cell density to $(1～10) \times 10^6$ cells/ml.

（5）将上述细胞悬液分装入冻存管中，拧紧冻存管盖子，标注清楚细胞名称、冻存日期等。

Equally divide the cell suspension into several cryogenic tubes and securely tighten their lids. Clearly write the cell name and the date of freezing on each tube.

（6）置 4℃ 普通冰箱中预冷 30 min。

Pre-cool the tubes for 30 min in a 4℃ refrigerator.

（7）将冻存管放入冻存盒中，立即转移入－80℃ 超低温冰箱过夜。

Place the cryogenic tubes into a freezing container and transfer it immediately into a－80℃ ultra-low temperature refrigerator overnight.

（8）次日将冻存管转移入液氮罐中，在记录本上记录清楚冻存管的位置、名称等信息。

The next day，transfer the cryogenic tubes to a liquid nitrogen tank. The location and name of the cell cryogenic tubes should be clearly recorded in a book.

（三）注意事项 Notes

（1）冻存细胞的生长状态要好，最好选择对数生长期的细胞。培养瓶中细胞密度不宜过高，并且在冻存前 24 h 内对培养基进行更换。

The growth state of the cells selected for cryopreservation should be good. It is best to select cells in logarithmic growth phase, and change the medium within 24 hours prior to cryopreservation. The density of cells in culture flask should not be too high before freezing.

(2) 冻存液的配方可根据细胞种类不同进行适当的调整,血清的浓度可以更高一些,甘油和 DMSO 的浓度也可在 5%～20%之间调整。

The formulation of the cryopreservation solution can be appropriately adjusted according to the cell type and the serum concentration can be higher than that used during cell culture. The concentration of glycerol and DMSO can also be adjusted between 5% and 20%.

(3) 最好在冻存后的数天里任意选取一支所冻存的细胞进行复苏,用以鉴定冻存效果。

It is best to select a sample of frozen cells for resuscitation within a few days after cryopreservation to identify the possible problems resulting from freezing.

(4) DMSO 不需要高压灭菌。此外,常温下 DMSO 对人体有害,应戴手套操作。

It is not necessary to sterilize DMSO under high pressure before using for cryopreservation. In addition, DMSO is harmful to human body at room temperature and should be handled using gloves.

(5) 不宜将冻存细胞放置在 0 ～— 60℃ 的温度范围过久,低温损伤主要发生在此温度区域。

It is not advisable to place frozen cells in the temperature range of 0 to−60℃ for too long. Low temperature damage mainly occurs in this temperature range.

(6) 冻存细胞的封口一定要紧。否则细胞冻存管可能会漏入液氮,再次取出时,导致冻存管爆炸。将冻存管放入液氮罐时,应防止被溅出的液氮冻伤。

Frozen cells must be sealed tightly. Otherwise, liquid nitrogen may leak into the cell cryogenic tube, possibly causing the tube to explode when brought to room temperature! Care should also be taken to avoid splashing the liquid nitrogen onto unprotected skin when placing cryogenic tubes into the liquid nitrogen tank.

(7) 为保证冻存效果,选择最佳的降温程序和速度也很重要。目前,多采用分段降温法,即利用不同温级的冰箱或液氮储存罐,将活细胞在不同的温度段分段降温冷却。例如,从室温降至 4℃,再依次降至 — 40℃、— 80℃、— 196℃(在各温度段维持时间视细胞的类型而定),一般以每分钟下降 1～10℃ 的速度为宜。

To ensure the proper freezing, it is important to choose the best cooling procedure and speed. At present, the stepwise cooling method is most often used, that is, using refrigerators, freezers and liquid nitrogen storage tanks to cool living cells during different temperature stages, such as from room temperature to 4℃, then to−40℃, next to−80℃ and finally to−196℃. Depending on the type of cells, generally good results are obtained at rates of temperature decreases of 1 to 10℃ per minute during each cooling stage.

二、细胞的复苏 Thawing of cells

（一）仪器与试剂 Required equipment and reagents

水浴锅、超净台、离心机、离心管、培养瓶、细胞培养箱、倒置显微镜、吸管、废液缸、细胞培养基和70%乙醇浸过的棉球等。

water bath, centrifuge, centrifuge tube, culture flask, cell culture incubator, inverted microscope, straw, waste tank, cell culture medium, 70% ethanol-impregnated cotton balls.

（二）操作步骤 Protocols

（1）准备工作：开启恒温水浴锅，将温度调节在45℃。

Preparation: Turn on the constant temperature water bath and adjust the temperature to 45℃.

（2）从液氮罐中取出冻存管，立即放入水浴锅中摇晃，快速融化冻存液。

Remove the cryogenic tube from the liquid nitrogen tank and immediately shake it by hand in the water bath to quickly melt the frozen solution.

（3）用乙醇棉球擦洗冻存管外部以降低污染机会。

Wash the outside of the cryogenic tube with an ethanol cotton ball to reduce the chance of contamination.

（4）在超净台内打开冻存管，将冻存液转移到预先加入有培养基的离心管中，700～800 r/min离心5 min。

Open the cryogenic tube, transfer the frozen solution to the centrifuge tube containing previously added culture medium and centrifuge at 700 to 800 r/min for 5 minutes.

（5）小心弃掉上清液，加入5 ml左右培养液重悬细胞。

Carefully remove and discard the supernatant and resuspend the cells in 5 ml of culture medium.

（6）将所得细胞悬液转移入培养瓶中，置于细胞培养箱培养。

Transfer the cell suspension into a culture flask, secure the flask cap and culture in the cell culture incubator.

（三）注意事项 Notes

（1）冻存液融化要迅速，使之迅速通过细胞最易受损的－5～0℃，细胞活力受损不大。

The cryopreservation solution should be rapidly thawed to allow the cells to quickly pass through the temperature range of －5 to 0℃, where the cells are most vulnerable to damage.

（2）离心速度不宜太高，避免对细胞的损伤。

To avoid damaging the cells, centrifugal speeds should not be too high.

（贺　颖）

第三章　亚细胞器和亚细胞结构的分离
Isolation of subcellular organelles and structures

细胞由各种亚细胞结构组成。其重要的研究手段之一是分离纯化亚细胞组分,观察它们的结构或进行生化分析。离心技术是实现这一目标的基本手段。一般认为,转速为10～30 Kr/min 的离心机称为高速离心机;转速超过 30 Kr/min 的离心机称为超速离心机。目前超速离心机的最高转速可达 150 Kr/min。

A cell is composed of various subcellular structures. One of the important research approaches is to isolate and purify subcellular components to observe their structures or perform biochemical analyses. Centrifugation is the basic techniques to achieve this goal.

第一节 ◉ 亚细胞器的分离
Isolation of subcellular organelles

分离亚细胞组分的第一步是制备组织匀浆或细胞匀浆。匀浆(homogenization)是指在低温条件下,将组织或细胞放在匀浆器中加入等渗匀浆介质(即 0.25 mol/L 蔗糖 — 0.003 mol/L 氯化钙溶液)研磨,使细胞被机械地研碎成为各种亚细胞组分和包含物的混合物。

The first step is to prepare tissue or cell homogenates. Homogenization is a process in which tissue or cells are placed in a homogenizer at low temperature and homogenized in homogenizing medium (i.e, 0.25 mol/L sucrose — 0.003 mol/L calcium chloride solution), so that the cells are mechanically separated into a mixture of various subcellular components and inclusions.

分离亚细胞组分的第二步是分级分离。通过低速到高速离心技术,使非均一混合体中的颗粒按大小轻重分批沉降到离心管的不同部位,再分部收集,即可得到各种亚细胞组分。由于样品中各种大小和密度不同的颗粒在离心开始时是均匀分布于整个离心管中的,故每级分离得到的第一次沉淀物必然不是纯的最重的颗粒,须经反复悬浮和离心加以纯化。分离亚细胞组分的主要离心技术是差速离心和密度梯度离心。

The second step is fractional separation. By centrifuging at various speeds, from low to high, subcellular particles in heterogeneous mixtures can be deposited on different parts of the centrifuge tube according to their size and weight, and then collected to obtain various subcellular components. Since the first precipitations obtained from each stage of separation do not necessarily include only the heaviest particles，the precipitated fractions must be repeatedly resuspended and centrifuged to allow purification. Both differential centrifugation and density gradient centrifugation are used to separate subcellular components.

　　差速离心（differential centrifugation）是在密度均一的介质中由低速到高速逐级离心，用于分离不同大小的细胞和细胞器。在差速离心中细胞器沉降的顺序依次为：细胞核、线粒体、溶酶体与过氧化物酶体、内质网与高尔基复合体，最后为核糖体。由于各种细胞器在大小和密度上相互重叠，一般重复 2～3 次效果较好。通过差速离心可将细胞器初步分离，但常需进一步通过密度梯度离心再行分离纯化。

　　Differential centrifugation involves differentially precipitating material at different speeds from a medium with uniform density. It is used to separate cells and organelles of different sizes. The sizes of cellular organelles in descending orders are：nuclei，mitochondria，lysosomes and peroxisomes，endoplasmic reticulum and the Golgi complex，and ribosomes. It is best to repeat differential centrifugations 2 to 3 times to avoid cross-contamination of components. Organelles can be separated preliminarily by differential centrifugation prior to further purification using density gradient centrifugation.

　　密度梯度离心（density gradient centrifugation）是用一定的介质在离心管内形成一连续或不连续的密度梯度，将细胞混悬液或匀浆置于介质的顶部，通过重力或离心力场的作用使细胞分层、分离。该方法常用的介质为氯化铯、蔗糖和多聚蔗糖。分离活细胞的介质要求：能产生密度梯度，且密度高时，黏度不高；pH 中性或易调为中性 pH 值；浓度大时渗透压不大；对细胞无毒。这类分离又可分为速度沉降和等密度沉降两种。速度沉降（velocity sedimentation）主要用于分离密度相近而大小不等的细胞或细胞器。这种方法所采用的介质密度较低，介质的最大密度应小于被分离生物颗粒的最小密度。生物颗粒（细胞或细胞器）在十分平缓的密度梯度介质中按各自的沉降系数以不同的速度沉降而达到分离。等密度沉降（isopycnic sedimentation）适用于分离密度不等的颗粒。细胞或细胞器在连续梯度的介质中经足够大离心力和足够长时间则沉降或漂浮到与自身密度相等的介质处，并停留在那里达到平衡，从而将不同密度的细胞或细胞器分离。等密度沉降通常在较高密度的介质中进行。介质的最高密度应大于被分离组分的最大密度。再者，这种方法所需要的力场通常比速度沉降法大 10～100 倍，故往往需要高速或超速离心，离心时间也较长。大的离心力、长的离心时间都对细胞不利。因此，这种方法适于分离细胞器，而不太适于分离和纯化细胞。

　　Density gradient centrifugation is a process in which a specific medium is used to form a continuous or discontinuous density gradient along the length of the centrifugation tubes. Cell suspensions or homogenates are placed on the top of the medium. During centrifugation，cells or components of the homogenates precipitate at different rates depending upon their shape and size or form distinct layers within the centrifugation tube at their intrinsic buoyant densities within the density gradient of medium established by the centrifugal force field. Cesium chloride，sucrose and polysucrose are commonly used as media in this method. The requirements of media for the separation of living cells include: the ability to produce a density gradient when centrifuged; low viscosity at high densities; intrinsically pH neutral or easily adjusted to neutral pH; low osmotic pressure at high concentrations; lack of toxicity to cells. Centrifugation methods can be divided into two kinds: velocity sedimentation and isopycnic sedimentation. Velocity sedimentation is mainly used to separate cells and organelles of similar density and unequal size. In the medium with lower density, the biological particles precipitate at different speeds according to their respective sedimentation coefficients. Isopycnic sedimentation applies to separating particles of unequal density. The cell or organelle in the continuous gradient medium will sink or float to the medium with the same density as itself after enough centrifugal force and enough time, and stay there to reach the equilibrium, so as to separate the cell or organelle with different density. This method requires larger centrifugal force and longer centrifugal time, so it is not suitable for cell separation, and is often used to separate organelles.

分离亚细胞组分的第三步是对分级分离得到的组分进行分析和确认。常用的方法包括形态和功能鉴定。

The third step is to analyze the components obtained by fractional separation for confirmation. Common analytical methods include morphological and functional identification.

第二节 ◎ 细胞核与线粒体的分离
Isolation of nucleus and mitochondria

一、仪器与试剂 Required equipment and reagents

玻璃匀浆器、普通离心机、台式高速离心机、普通天平、光学显微镜、离心管、吸管、0.25 mol/L 蔗糖－0.003 mol/L 氯化钙溶液、1%甲苯胺蓝染液、0.02%詹纳斯绿 B 染液、0.9%氯化钠溶液。

Glass homogenizer, ordinary centrifuge, high-speed centrifuge, ordinary balance, light microscope, centrifuge tubes, pipettes, 0.25 mol/L sucrose－0.003 mol/L $CaCl_2$ solution, 1% toluidine blue dye solution, 0.02% Janus green B dye solution, 0.9% NaCl solution.

二、操作步骤 Protocols

(一) 制备肝组织匀浆 Preparation of liver homogenate
(1) 将 BALB/c 小鼠用颈椎脱臼法处死,迅速打开腹腔取出肝脏,剪成小块(去除结缔组织)尽快置于盛有 0.9%氯化钠的烧杯中,反复洗涤,除去血污,用滤纸吸去表面的液体。

Sacrifice BALB/c mice by cervical dislocation, cut open its abdomen and remove its liver. The liver is cut into small pieces (removing connective tissue) and placed in a beaker containing 0.9% NaCl as soon as possible. After repeated washing, remove blood and the surface liquid by blotting with filter paper.

（2）称取 1 g 肝组织（湿重）放在平皿中，用量筒量取 8 ml 预冷的 0.25 mol/L 蔗糖－0.003 mol/L 氯化钙溶液，先加少量该溶液于平皿中，尽量剪碎肝组织后，再全加入。

Weigh out 1 g of liver tissue (wet weight) and place in a dish. Prepare 8 ml precooled 0.25 mol/L sucrose － 0.003 mol/L $CaCl_2$ solution. Add a small amount of this solution to the dish and cut the liver tissue into as small pieces as possible and add the rest of solution.

（3）剪碎的肝组织倒入匀浆管中，使匀浆管下端浸入盛有冰块的烧杯中。一手持匀浆管，一手将匀浆捣杆垂直插入匀浆管中，研磨 3～5 次。用 8 层纱布（先用蔗糖液湿润）过滤匀浆液于离心管中，然后制备涂片①，做好标记，自然干燥。

Put the mixture of liver fragments and solution into homogenate tube，immersing the bottom of homogenate tube in a beaker containing ice cubes. With one hand hold homogenate tube，used the other hand to insert the homogenate rod vertically into homogenate tube，grinding the tissue 3 to 5 times. Filter the mixture into a centrifuge tube through 8 layers of gauze (wetting with sucrose solution first). Make a smear of the homogenate on a glass slide. Label this as slide ① and allow it to dry in the air.

（二）分级分离　Fractionation

1. 细胞核的分离提取　Isolation of nuclei

（1）将装有滤液的离心管配平后，放入普通离心机，以 2 500 r/min，离心 15 min；缓缓取上清液，移入放在冰块中的高速离心管内，待分离线粒体用；同时涂一张上清液片②，做好标记，自然干燥；余下的沉淀物进行下一步骤。

After balancing the centrifuge tube containing the filtrate and centrifuge the sample at 2 500 r/min for 15 min. Transfer the supernatant to a high-speed centrifugal tube carefully，and temporarily store on ice for isolation of mitochondria. Make a smear of the supernatant on another glass slide，label this as slide ② and let it dry in the air.

（2）用 6 ml 0.25 mol/L 蔗糖－0.003 mol/L 氯化钙溶液悬浮沉淀物，2 500 r/min 离心 15 min 弃上清液，将残留液体用吸管吹打成悬液，滴一滴于干净的载玻片上，即涂片③，自然干燥。

Resuspend the pellet from the centrifugation in 6 ml 0.25 mol/L sucrose-0.003 mol/L $CaCl_2$ solution and centrifuge again at 2 500 r/min for 15 min. Discard the supernatant. Resuspend the pellet with the residual liquid and use this to make a third smear on a new glass slide，label slide ③ and let it dry in the air.

（3）将涂片①、②、③用 1% 甲苯胺蓝染色后盖片，显微镜视下观察。

Stain the three slides (①,②,③) with 1% toluidine blue, and observe differences among these slides under light microscope.

2. 线粒体的分离提取　Isolation of mitochondria

（1）将上述装有上清液的高速离心管，从装有冰块的烧杯中取出，配平后，以 17 000 r/min 离心 20 min，弃上清液，留取沉淀物。加入 0.25 mol/L 蔗糖－0.003 mol/L 氯化钙溶液 1 ml，用吸管吹打成悬液，以 17 000 r/min 离心 20 min，将上清液吸入另一试管中，留取沉淀物。

Remove the high-speed centrifugal tube containing supernatant from the first centrifugation from the beaker containing ice cubes，balance it and centrifuge at 17 000 r/min for 20 min. Discard the supernatant and add 1 ml 0. 25 mol/L sucrose — 0.003 mol/L $CaCl_2$ solution to the centrifuge tube and use a pipette to resuspend the pellet. Centrifuge the sample at 17 000 r/min for 20 min transfer the supernatant to centrifuge tube and retain the pellet.

（2）加入 0.25 mol/L 蔗糖—0.003 mol/L 氯化钙溶液 0.1 ml 混匀成悬液。取上清液和沉淀悬液，分别滴一滴于干净载玻片上（分别标记为④、⑤涂片），各滴一滴 0.02%詹纳斯绿 B 染液，盖上盖片染色 20 min。

Add 0.1 ml 0.25 mol/L sucrose-0.003 mol/L $CaCl_2$ solution and mix it into suspension. Drop one drop of supernatant and pellet on clean glass slides（mark the slides ④ and ⑤ respectively），and stain them by one drop containing 0.02% Janus green B for 20 min.

（3）油镜下观察，颗粒状的线粒体被詹纳斯绿 B 染成蓝绿色。

When viewed under a microscope using an oil objective lens，the granular mitochondria are stained blue-green by Janus green B.

三、附录   Appendix

（一）Ringer 液   Ringer's solution

NaCl	0.9 g
KCl	0.042 g
$CaCl_2$	0.025 g
Purified water	100 ml

（二）1/300 詹纳斯绿 B 染液   1/300 Janus green B dye solution

取詹纳斯绿 1 g，加 Ringer 液 300 ml。现用现配。

Add 1 g of Janus green B to 300 ml of Ringer's solution. Use immediately after preparation.

（三）0.25 mol/L 蔗糖—0.003 mol/L 氯化钙溶液   0.25 mol/L sucrose — 0.003 mol/L $CaCl_2$ solution

Sucrose	85.5 g
$CaCl_2$	0.33 g
Purified water	1 000 ml

第三节 ◉ 微粒体和溶酶体的分离
Separation of microsomes and lysosomes

一、微粒体的分离   Separation of microsomes

细胞通过匀浆破碎时，细胞质膜碎成片段，这些膜片段的末端融合形成直径<100 nm 的

小泡。来自不同细胞器(细胞核、线粒体、质膜、内质网等)的小泡有不同的特性,所以可以将这些小泡相互分离。由内膜系统衍生而来的小膜泡形成相似大小的膜泡异质性集合体,称微粒体(microsome)。分离微粒体的方法是利用分级离心方法,去掉细胞核、线粒体后,经超速离心法而制备。

When cells are homogenized，the cytoplasmic membrane is broken into fragments，the edges of which fuse to form into vesicles of less than 100 nm in diameter. These vesicles are distinct from vesicles derived from intracellular organelles （nucleus，mitochondria，cell membrane，endoplasmic reticulum，etc.）. Vesicles that have different characteristics can be physically separated. Microsomes are similar sized，heterogeneous aggregates of membrane vesicles derived from intracellular organelles. These can also be isolated by fractional separation. After removing nuclei and mitochondria, microsomes can be isolated using ultracentrifugation.

具体步骤如下。

The required steps are as follows.

(1) 将体重约为 300 g 饥饿 20 h 后的大鼠断头,取出肝脏,洗涤,剪碎,加 2 倍体积的介质溶液(含 0.15 mol/L 蔗糖,0.025 mol/L KCl,0.1 mol/L Tris - HCl pH 7.4,0.005 mol/L $MgCl_2$),在玻璃匀浆器中匀浆。

Sacrifice a rat with a body weight of about 300 g that had been deprived food for 20 hours. Remove the liver，wash and cut it into pieces. Add twice the volume of the medium solution (containing 0.15 mol/L sucrose，0.025 mol/L KCl，0.1 mol/L Tris - HCl pH 7.4 and 0.005 mol/L $MgCl_2$) to liver and homogenize the mixture in a glass homogenizer.

(2) 15 000×g 离心 10 min,弃沉淀物,取上清液。

Centrifuge 15 000×g for 10 minutes, discard the pellet and retain the supernatant.

(3) 100 000×g 离心 60 min,弃上清液,取沉淀物,沉淀物即为微粒体。

Centrifuge 100 000×g for 60 minutes，discard the supernatant and retain the pellet (microsomes).

(4) 将微粒体保存在介质溶液中。

Store the microsomes in a medium solution.

二、溶酶体的分离　Separation of lysosomes

溶酶体是由一层单位膜包围,内含多种酸性水解酶的泡状结构。溶酶体含有 40 多种水解酶,其中包括蛋白酶、核酸降解酶和糖苷酶等。其主要功能是对细胞内物质的消化作用。此外溶酶体与器官形成、激素分泌的调节以及某些疾病的发生密切相关。可采用如下方法分离获得。

Lysosomes are vesicular structures surrounded by single membrane that contain a variety of acidic hydrolytic enzymes. Lysosomes contain more than 40 kinds of hydrolytic enzymes，including proteases，nucleic acid degrading enzymes and glycosidases. Their main function is the digestion of intracellular substances. In addition, lysosomes play important roles in organ formation, regulation of hormone secretion and liability to some diseases. Lysosomes can be isolated using the following method.

（1）制备蔗糖梯度溶液：取带有两个小杯的梯度混合器，两个小杯分别装入 117 ml 2.1 mol/L 蔗糖和 13 ml 1.1 mol/L 的蔗糖。

Prepare a sucrose gradient solution using a gradient mixer with two small cups, loaded with 117 ml 2.1 mol/L sucrose and 13 ml 1.1 mol/L sucrose, respectively.

（2）将大鼠处死取出肾脏，以 1∶8（重量/体积）比例加入 0.3 mol/L 蔗糖，然后在玻璃匀浆器中匀浆肾脏组织。

Sacrifice a rat and remove its kidneys. Add sucrose solution (0.3 mol/L) at a ratio of 1∶8 (weight/volume) and homogenize the kidney tissue in a glass homogenizer.

（3）150×g 离心 10 min，弃沉淀物，取上清液。9 000×g 再离心 3 min，弃上清液，取沉淀物。

Centrifuged the homogenate at 150×g for 10 minutes. Discard the pellet and retain the supernatant. Centrifuge the supernatant at 9 000×g for 3 minutes. Discard the supernatant and retain the pellet.

（4）沉淀物从上至下依次为白色、黄褐色、暗褐色 3 种不同颜色层，上层为膜成分的混合物，中层为线粒体部分，最底层则为半纯化的溶酶体。先用吸管小心吸掉上层，然后沿管壁加入几毫升 0.3 mol/L 蔗糖，慢慢摇管使中间层悬浮起来弃之。用 0.3 mol/L 蔗糖洗涤 1 次，底层溶酶体部分悬浮在 2.5 ml 0.3 mol/L 蔗糖中。

The pellet comprises 3 layers with different colors: white, yellowish brown and dark brown (top to bottom). The upper layer contains a mixture of membrane components, the middle layer contains mitochondria, and the bottom layer contains semi-purified lysosomes. Carefully remove the upper layer using a pipette, then add a few milliliters of 0.3 mol/L sucrose along the wall of the tube and slowly shake the tube to resuspend the exposed middle (mitochondrial) layer. Discard the resuspended mitochondrial layer. Repeat this procedure one more time with 0.3 mol/L sucrose to remove the residual mitochondrial layer. Gently resuspend the bottom (lysosomal) layer in 2.5 ml 0.3 mol/L sucrose.

（5）将 2 ml 悬浮的半纯化的溶酶体铺在蔗糖梯度上面，用玻璃棒搅动最上层的梯度，使梯度和溶酶体之间的界面破坏，然后 100 000×g 离心 150 min。离心结果可见：梯度溶液分 3 条明显的带和较少的沉淀物。最下层的暗黄色到褐色的带即为纯化的溶酶体。以上所有操作需在 0～4℃下进行。

Load 2 ml of the resuspended, semi-purified lysosomes onto the sucrose gradient, and stir the uppermost gradient with a glass rod to break the interface between the gradient and the lysosomes. Centrifuge the sample at 100 000×g for 150 minutes. Centrifugation reveals a gradient solution divided into three distinct bands and containing little pellet. The lowest layer, containing bands of dark yellow to brown, contain purified lysosomes. All these operations should be carried out at 0 to 4℃.

第四节 ⊙ 细胞总蛋白质的分离提取
Separation and extraction of total cell protein

细胞器是一种动态的结构,如内质网、细胞核和高尔基复合体等,其蛋白质组成除了驻留蛋白质之外,还包括穿梭蛋白质和瞬间相互作用的蛋白质。对于这些组成成分的研究,即亚细胞蛋白质组研究将有助于对这些蛋白质做全面的挖掘,从而对细胞器的功能作深入阐述。蛋白质提取与制备的具体操作方法如下。

Intracellular organelles, such as the endoplasmic reticulum, nucleus and Golgi complex, are dynamic structures that contain not only resident proteins, but also proteins that shuttle through the organelle or transiently interact with its resident proteins. The identification and study of resident and non-resident proteins yield important insights concerning the functions of intracellular organelles. Specific methods for protein extraction and preparation are as follows.

一、材料的选择 Material selection

材料的选择主要依据实验目的而定。一般要注意种属的关系,提前查阅制备的难易情况。

The choice of starting materials depends mainly on experimental goals. In general, we should pay attention to differences between species and assess potential experimental difficulties in advance.

二、蛋白质的分离 Separation of protein

(一)细胞的破碎 Breaking cells

对细胞内及多细胞生物组织中蛋白质的分离提取均须先将细胞破碎,使蛋白质充分释放到溶液中。不同生物体或同一生物体的不同组织,其细胞破坏难易不一,使用方法也不完全相同。如动物胰、肝、脑组织一般较为柔软,普通匀浆器研磨即可;而肌肉及心脏组织较韧,需预先绞碎后再进行匀浆。

To extract proteins from cells or multicellular biological tissues, cells must be broken to release their contents into solution. Different organisms and different tissues of the same organism have different difficulties with respect to breaking cell. Different methods can be used for different tissues. For example, pancreas, liver and brain tissues are generally soft, allowing the use of ordinary homogenizers. By contrast, muscle and heart tissues are tough, and need to be mechanically or physically broken up prior to homogenization.

1. 机械方法 Mechanical methods

主要通过机械切力的作用使组织细胞破碎。常用器械有:①高速组织捣碎机(转速可达 10 000 r/min,具有高速转动的锋利刀片),宜用于动物内脏组织的破碎;②玻璃匀浆器(用两个磨砂面相互摩擦,将细胞磨碎),适用于少量材料,也可用不锈钢或硬质塑料等制成。小量的组织可用研钵与适当的缓冲剂磨碎提取,也可加氧化铝、石英砂及玻璃粉磨细。但在磨细时局部往往生热导致变性或 pH 值显著变化,尤其是用玻璃粉和氧化铝时。此外,磨细剂的吸附也可导致蛋白质损失。

Mechanical methods are used to break tissue cells through shear force. Commonly used instruments include:①high-speed tissue cutting machines (blenders) with high-sharp blades at rotate at up to10 000 r/min are used for animal visceral tissue;②Homogenizers made of glass, stainless steel or plastic are suitable for breaking up a small amounts of tissue. Mortars and pestles can also be used for breaking small amounts of tissue suspended in appropriate buffers, with possible addition of alumina, fine quartz sand or glass powder to facilitate the breakdown of tough materials. Mortars and pestles, however, are not always an appropriate choice, since the heat generated by grinding may lead to significant protein denaturation and pH changes, especially when using glass powder and alumina. In addition, grinding agents often absorb proteins leading to loss of starting material.

2. 物理方法　Physical methods

主要通过各种物理因素的作用,使组织细胞破碎。①反复冻融法:将组织细胞置于 −20℃ 或 以下使之冰冻,然后再缓慢地融解。如此反复操作数次,因细胞内冰晶的形成及细胞内外溶剂浓度的突然改变而破坏细胞结构。②急热骤冷法:将材料投入沸水中数分钟,然后立即置于冰浴中使之迅速冷却,绝大部分细胞可被破坏。③超声波法:暴露于 9～10 千兆声波或 10～500 千兆超声波所产生的机械振动中,此法方便且效果好,但一次处理量较小。应用超声波处理时应注意避免溶液中气泡的存在。处理一些超声波敏感的蛋白酶时慎用。④加压破碎法:通过加一定的气压或水压使细胞破碎。

Physical methods break tissue cells mainly through the effects of various non-mechanical effects. ① Repeated freezing and thawing method:the cellular structures are destroyed due to the formation of intracellular ice crystals and the sudden changes of solvent concentrations inside and outside the cell. ② Rapid heating and rapid cooling method:put samples into boiling water for a few minutes, and then put them in an ice bath to cool down rapidly. Most cells are destroyed. ③ Ultrasonic method:expose samples to vibrations produced by 9 to 10 gigabit sound waves or 10 to 500 gigabit ultrasonic. This method is convenient and effective. Most suitable for small samples. Precautions:avoid creating bubbles in the sample;not suitable for the study of ultrasound sensitive protein. ④ Pressure method:subject samples to high air or water pressure to break cells open.

3. 化学及生物化学方法　Chemical and biochemical methods

①化学渗透法:某些有机溶剂(如丙酮等)、表面活性剂[如十二烷基硫酸钠(SDS)、氯化十二烷基吡啶及去氧胆酸钠等]、低渗缓冲液、金属螯合剂等化学药品可以改变细胞膜或细胞壁的通透性,从而使细胞内含物有选择性地渗透出来。②自溶法:在一定 pH 值和适当的温度下,利用自身的蛋白酶将细胞破坏,使细胞内含物释放出来。自体溶解时需要时间,需加少量甲苯、氯仿等。注意防止污染。因该过程中 pH 值变化显著,要随时调节 pH 值。因自溶时间较长,不易控制,所以制备活性蛋白质时慎用。③酶溶法:此法多适用于细菌和其他微生物,应用各种水解

酶,如溶菌酶、纤维素酶、蜗牛酶、脂酶等,将细胞裂解,使细胞内含物释放出来。

Chemical and biochemical methods include: ① Chemical osmosis method: some organic solvents (such as acetone), surfactants (such as sodium dodecyl sulfate, dodecylpyridinium chloride and sodium deoxycholate), low permeability buffers and metal chelating agents can change the permeability of cell membranes or cell walls, stimulating the selective release of certain cell inclusions. ② Autolysis method: at a certain pH and temperatures proteases within the cell are activated, resulting the damage to the cell membrane and the release of cellular contents. Autolysis takes place slowly and may require the addition of small amounts of toluene, chloroform or other solvents, which require special handling or disposal. The pH should be continuously monitored and, if required, adjusted to maintain an appropriate pH. Autolysis takes a long time and is not easy to control, and therefore may not be suitable for the isolation of some enzymes or proteins. ③ Enzymolysis method: this method is applicable to bacteria and other microorganisms. Various hydrolytic enzymes or mixtures of enzymes, including lysozyme, cellulase, lipase and snailase, are used to break down cell walls and release cellular contents.

(二) 细胞器蛋白的分离　Separation of organelle proteins

为制备和纯化某一特定细胞器上的生物大分子,防止其他细胞组分的干扰,细胞破碎后常将细胞内各组分先行分离。各类生物大分子在细胞内的分布是不同的,因此制备细胞器上的生物大分子时,预先需要对整个细胞结构和各类生物大分子在细胞内分布有所了解。

To prepare and purify biomacromolecules from a specific organelle and prevent interference from other cellular components, intracellular components are usually separated first after cell fragmentation. The distribution of all kinds of biomacromolecules in cells is different. Therefore, the whole cell structure and the distribution of all kinds of biomacromolecules in cells must be understood in advance.

细胞经过破碎后,在适当介质中进行差速离心。利用细胞各组分质量大小不同,沉降于离心管内不同的层,分离后即得所需组分。细胞器的分离制备,介质的选择十分重要。一般选用蔗糖、Ficoll(一种蔗糖多聚物)或葡萄糖-聚乙二醇等高分子溶液。大部分蛋白质均溶于水、稀盐、稀碱或稀酸溶液中。因此,蛋白质的提取一般以水为主。稀盐溶液和缓冲溶液对蛋白质稳定性好、溶度大,也是提取蛋白质最常用的溶剂。

After breaking cells, differential centrifugation is carried out in an appropriate medium. The components are deposited in different layers of the centrifuge tube based on different mass sizes. The selection of medium is very important. Generally, sucrose, Ficoll (a kind of polysucrose) or glucose-polyethylene glycol and other polymer solutions are selected. Most proteins are soluble in water, dilute salts, dilute bases or dilute acids. Therefore, protein extraction is generally based on water. Dilute salt solution and buffer solution have good stability and solubility for protein, and are also the most commonly used solvent for protein extraction

（刘　丹）

第四章　基于抗体的细胞化学显示

Antibody-based cytochemistry

在生命科学研究领域,抗体已被成功地应用于捕获靶分子(抗原)、亲和层析纯化蛋白、组织细胞中靶分子定位研究等诸多方向。这些技术是基于抗体与抗原发生特异性结合的特性,主要可分为 4 种类型:①利用抗体"示踪"靶分子;②利用抗体捕获靶分子;③利用抗体进行蛋白功能学研究;④通过和芯片技术的结合用于蛋白表达谱研究。

In the field of life sciences, antibodies have been successfully applied to capture target molecules (antigens), purified proteins by affinity chromatography, and target molecule localization in tissue cells. These techniques are based on the specific binding of antibodies to antigens and can be divided into four types: ①Using antibodies to "trace" target molecules; ②Using antibodies to capture target molecules; ③Using Antibodies to study protein function; ④Combination of antibody and chip-technology to study protein expression profile.

第一节 ◎ 抗体的标记
Antibody labeling

在绝大多数情况下,当抗体分子被应用于研究时均需被标记。依据实验目的不同,所采用的标记方法和标记物通常也不同。

In most cases, antibody molecules need to be labeled when used in research. Labeling methods and markers used are usually different depending on the purpose of the experiment.

一、抗体标记的直接法与间接法　The direct and indirect labeling of antibodies

(一) 直接法　Direct labeling

直接法是将纯化后的抗体先与标记物直接结合,然后再与靶分子(抗原)结合,通过检测抗体所携带的标记物来对靶分子(抗原)进行定性、定位、定量测量的方法。

Direct labeling involves directly linking a marker to purified antibodies, which are then used to bind a target molecule (antigen). The target molecule (antigen) can be localized and quantitatively measured by detecting the marker bound to the antibody.

（二）间接法 Indirect labeling

间接法与直接法不同,抗体既不需纯化,也不需标记,而是在抗体与相应靶分子(抗原)结合后,洗去未结合抗体,然后通过利用已标记好的第二抗体(二抗)与一抗的结合来间接标记出靶分子(抗原)的存在情况。

The indirect labeling is different from the direct labeling. In this method, antibodies do not need to be purified or labeled. Instead, after the antibodies are combined with the target molecule (antigen), the unbound antibodies are washed out, and the sample combined with labeled secondary antibodies that specifically bind the primary antibodies. In this way, target molecules (antigens) can be indirectly labeled.

二、标记物的选择 Choice of markers

无论是直接法还是间接法,标记物的选择至关重要。表4-1所列出的就是一些常用标记物及其相应的检测方法和优缺点等。

The choice of markers is very important, whether used in direct or indirect labeling methods. Table 4-1 lists some common markers and their corresponding detection methods, as well as their advantages and disadvantages.

表4-1 标记物的选择

标记物	检测方法	优点	缺点	应用
生物素	与各种标记物偶联的亲和素与链霉亲和素	保存时间长,灵敏度高,检测手段多样	步骤过多,存在内源性生物素干扰,有些底物对人体有害	免疫组织化学、免疫印迹
荧光素	荧光显微镜或荧光计	保存时间长,分辨率高	自发荧光,易淬灭	免疫组织化学
酶	底物显色	保存时间长,灵敏度高,肉眼直接可见,检测手段多样	步骤过多,存在内源性酶的干扰,分辨率低,有些底物对人体有害	免疫组织化学、免疫印迹
^{125}I 或 ^{131}I	γ计数仪、放射自显影	易于直接标记,灵敏度高	半衰期短,对人体有害	免疫印迹,定性、定量免疫分析
生物合成	放射自显影、β计数仪	不损伤抗体,操作简便	半衰期短,敏感性低,需杂交瘤细胞	免疫印迹,定性、定量免疫分析
胶体金	显微镜、电子显微镜、肉眼	特异性强,灵敏度高,应用范围广,可用于双重和多重标记	对试剂、玻璃器皿的要求极高,标记物浓度较高	免疫组织化学、流式细胞术,定性、定量免疫分析

Table 4-1 Choice of markers

Markers	Detection methods	Advantages	Disadvantages	Application
Biotin	Avidin and streptavidin coupled with various markers	Long storage time, high sensitivity and various detection methods	Too many steps, interference from endogenous biotin, some substrates harmful to human health	Immunohistochemistry, Western blotting

Markers	Detection methods	Advantages	Disadvantages	Application
Fluorescent pigment	Fluorescence microscopy or fluorimeter	Long storage time, high resolution	Spontaneous fluorescence, easily quenched	Immunohistochemistry
Enzyme	chromogenic substrate assay	Long storage time, high sensitivity, macroscopic and various detection methods	Too many steps, endogenous biotin interference, low resolution, some substrates are harmful to human health	Immunohistochemistry, Western blotting
^{125}I or ^{131}I	γ counter, autoradiography	Direct labeling, high sensitivity	Short half-life, harmful to human health	Western blotting, qualitative and quantitative immunoassay
biosynthesis	Autoradiography, β counter	Does not damage the antibody, simple operation	Short half-life, low sensitivity, need hybridoma cells	Western blotting, qualitative and quantitative immunoassay
colloidal gold	Light microscope, electron microscope, unaided eye	High specificity, high sensitivity, wide range of applications, can be used for double and multiple tagging	High requirements for reagents and glassware, high concentration of markers	Immunohistochemistry, flow cytometry, qualitative and quantitative immunoassay

第二节 ◎ 免疫组织（细胞）化学技术
Immunohistochemistry and immunocytochemistry

　　免疫组织化学技术（immunohistochemistry，IHC）或免疫细胞化学技术（immunocytochemistry，ICC）是用经标记的特异性抗体在组织或细胞原位通过特异性抗原抗体反应和化学的呈色反应，对相应抗原进行定性、定位、定量测定的一项技术。

　　Immunohistochemistry (IHC) or immunocytochemistry (ICC) involves using labeled antibodies that bind to specific antigens in tissues or cells *in situ*, allowing the locations and relative levels of the antigens to be visualized.

一、研究内容

　　免疫组织化学技术和免疫细胞化学技术将抗原抗体免疫反应的特异性、组织化学的可见性结合起来，借助显微镜(包括荧光显微镜、电子显微镜)的显像与放大作用，在细胞、亚细胞水平检测各种细胞组织成分，如蛋白质、多肽、核酸、部分类酯、多糖、激素、病原体(寄生虫、细菌、病毒)、受体、神经递质、肿瘤的标记物(抗原或相关抗原)等，是免疫学、病理生理学和蛋白质研究的重要技术手段。

IHC and ICC combine the specificity of antigen-antibody binding with the generation of visible signals (e. g., fluorescence or colored precipitated dyes) that mark the locations of target antigens. Used in combination with various kinds of microscopy (including fluorescence microscopy and electron microscopy) and amplification methods, the method allows the *in situ* detection of various components of tissues at cellular and subcellular levels. Targets suitable for detection using this method include, specific proteins, polypeptides, nucleic acids, esters, polysaccharides, hormones, pathogens (parasites, bacteria, viruses), receptors, neurotransmitters, and tumor markers (antigens or related antigens). For these reasons, this method has become an important technique in the fields of immunology, pathophysiology and protein research.

免疫组织（细胞）化学的全过程包括：①抗原的提取与纯化；②免疫动物或细胞融合，制备特异性抗体以及抗体的纯化；③将显色剂与抗体结合形成标记抗体；④组织细胞标本的制备；⑤免疫细胞化学反应及呈色反应；⑥结果的观察与分析。

IHC and ICC protocol include：①Extraction and purification of antigens；②Immunization of animals or fusion of cells to prepare specific antibodies and the purification of those antibodies；③Linking chromogenic agents to the antibodies to produce labeled antibodies；④Preparation of samples；⑤Carrying out immunocytochemical reactions and chromogenic reactions；⑥Observation and analysis of results.

二、标本的制备　Preparation of specimens

（一）标本的取材　Acquisition of specimens

1. 体细胞取材方法　Acquisition of somatic cells

（1）印片法：主要用于从活组织检查标本和手术切除标本中获取细胞。首先将标本剖开，最大限度暴露组织病变区，然后将载玻片轻压于病变组织区，吸附脱落的细胞。

Printing：This technique is primarily used to obtain cells from biopsy specimens and surgically excised specimens. First, cut the specimen to expose the lesion area, then lightly press a glass slide onto the surface of the lesion to absorb the exposed cells.

（2）穿刺取样涂片法：用细针穿刺从实质性器官（如软组织、肝、肾、脾、淋巴结和骨髓）的病变区吸取病变区的体液，然后进行涂片。

Puncture sampling smear：Use a fine-needle to puncture the lesion area within soft tissues, liver, kidney, spleen, lymph nodes, or bone marrow, and draw the tissue and fluid out of the lesion area and smear a small amount on a glass slide.

（3）体液涂片法：主要适用于胸腔积液、腹腔积液、尿液、脑脊液等含细胞较少的标本，先通过离心获取细胞沉淀物，经适当稀释后再进行涂片。

Body fluid smear：This method is particularly suitable for pleural effusions, ascites, urine, cerebrospinal fluid and other specimens containing few cells. First, concentrate the cells within the fluid by centrifugation, then resuspend the pelleted cells at an appropriate dilution, and smear a small amount on a glass slide.

2. 培养细胞取材方法 Acquisition of cultured cells

(1) 细胞爬片法：适合于贴附依赖型细胞。将干净(消毒处理)的盖玻片放置入培养液中,细胞便会自然贴附在其上。

Cell slide：It is suitable for attachment-dependent cells. When a clean (sterilized) cover slide is placed in the culture medium, the cells will naturally adhere to it.

(2) 涂片法：适合于悬浮生长的培养细胞。直接取悬浮生长的培养细胞或通过离心收集细胞,再经适当的洗涤和稀释后进行涂片。

Cell smear：It is suitable for suspended cultured cells. Suspended cultured cells are directly taken or collected by centrifugation, and then smeared after washing and dilution.

(3) 组织材料的获取：主要通过组织切片技术获得。根据包埋剂的不同可分为：冷冻切片、石蜡切片、塑料切片、超薄切片和碳蜡切片等类型。

Tissue acquisition：Tissue is primarily obtained by tissue slicing technique. Based on the type of embedding agent, tissues samples can be obtained from frozen sections, paraffin sections, plastic sections, ultrathin sections, or carbon wax section.

(二) 标本的固定 Fixation of specimens

固定的目的是为了更好地将细胞和组织的原有形态、结构及成分保留下来,让蛋白质变性,使内源性消化酶失活。对免疫组织化学和免疫细胞化学而言,可用的固定剂种类多样,性能也不尽相同,在使用时应注意考虑不同固定剂对抗原的影响,防止抗原的弥散以及活性的丢失。

The purpose of fixation is to preserve the original morphological structure and components of cells and tissues, while denaturing proteins and endogenous inactivating digestive enzymes. For IHC and ICC there are many kinds of fixatives available, each with different properties. When using fixatives, attention should be paid to the effects of different fixatives on antigens to prevent their delocalization and/or inactivation.

常见的固定剂有醛类(如10%的中性缓冲甲醛(福尔马林),4%的多聚甲醛等)、非醛类(如碳化二亚胺、对苯醌等)、丙酮及醇类固定剂。常见的固定方法有浸入法和灌注法等。

Common fixatives include：aldehydes (10% neutral buffer formalin, 4% polyformaldehyde, etc.), non-aldehydes (carbodiimide, p-benzoquinone, etc.), acetone and ethanol fixatives. Common fixation methods include immersion and perfusion.

三、免疫荧光技术 Immunofluorescence

免疫荧光技术(Immunofluorescence, IF)是利用抗原与抗体可发生特异性结合的原理,先将已知的抗原或抗体标记上荧光素,进而再利用这种荧光抗体(或抗原)去检查细胞或组织内的相应抗原(或抗体)。根据检测目的以及待检物的不同特点,免疫荧光技术有直接法、间接法、补体法、双重荧光标记法等不同形式。

Immunofluorescence (IF) is based on the principle of specific binding between antigens and antibodies：known antigens or antibodies are labeled with fluorescein, and then the fluorescent antibodies (or antigens) are used to detect the corresponding antigens (or antibodies) in cells or tissues.

（一）荧光抗体的制备　Preparation of fluorescent antibodies

常用的荧光素分子主要有异硫氰酸(fluorescein-5-isothiocyanate，FITC)、四乙基罗丹明(tetraethylrodamine B200，RB200)、四甲基罗丹明异硫氰酸酯(tetramethylrhodamine isothiocyanate，TRITC)、藻红蛋白(phycoerthrin，PE)等，它们在不同波长激发光的作用下可发出不同颜色的荧光。

The commonly used fluorescein derivatives include：fluorescein-5-isothiocyanate (FITC)，tetraethylrodamine B200 (RB200)，tetramethylrhodamine isothiocyanate (TRITC)，and phycoerthrin (PE). The molecules emit fluorescent light when illuminated by light of higher wavelengths.

1. 异硫氰酸荧光素标记抗体的制备　Preparation of FITC

（1）仪器与试剂 Required equipment and reagents：透析袋、紫外分光光度计、Sephadex G25 柱、纯化过的单克隆抗体或多克隆抗体、FITC、pH 9～9.5 的碳酸盐缓冲液、pH7.2 的磷酸盐缓冲液(phosphate buffer saline，PBS)、DMSO。

Dialysis bag，an ultraviolet spectrophotometer，Sephadex G25 column，purified monoclonal or polyclonal antibody，FITC，carbonate buffer (pH 9～9.5)，PBS (pH 7.2)，DMSO.

（2）操作步骤 Protocol

1）将纯化过的抗体放入透析袋中，在加有 pH 9.0～9.5 碳酸盐缓冲液的容器中透析过夜(4℃)，透析后抗体被转移到一小塑料管中备用。

Purified antibodies are put into a dialysis bag and dialyzed overnight at 4℃ in carbonate buffer (pH 9.0 to 9.5). After dialysis，the antibodies are transferred to small plastic tube for later use.

2）配制 FITC-DMSO 溶液：称取适量 FITC，加入 DMSO 溶解，使 FITC 终浓度保持在 1 mg/ml 左右。

Prepare FITC-DMSO solution：weigh appropriate amount of FITC，add DMSO to dissolve，ensure that the final concentration of FITC is about 1 mg/ml.

3）按照适当比例将 FITC-DMSO 溶液逐滴加到透析后的抗体溶液中。通常当抗体的浓度为 1 mg/ml 时，FITC 的加入量为 50 μg/ml；当抗体的浓度为 5～10 mg/ml 时，FITC 的加入量则降为 25 μg/ml。

Slowly add the FITC-DMSO solution to the antibody solution after dialysis. Usually，when the concentration of antibody is 1 mg/ml，the amount of FITC is 50 μg/ml；when the concentration of antibody is 5 to 10 mg/ml，the amount of FITC is reduced to 25 μg/ml.

4）将上述标记物用 PBS 稀释至 2.5 ml，室温下避光搅拌 2 h。

The above mixture is diluted to 2.5 ml with PBS and stirred for 2 hours at room temperature.

5）用 Sephadex G25 柱除去游离荧光素分子，收集第一个 PBS 洗脱峰(荧光素蛋白结合峰)，按照下式计算 F/P 值。

Load this mixture onto a Sephadex G25 column and elute with PBS to separate the fluorescein-labeled antibodies from free fluorescein-5-isothiocyanate/fluorescein. The first fluorescent elution peak contains the fluorescein-labeled antibodies，while the free fluorescein-5-isothiocyanate/fluorescein is retained in the column. Calculate the ratio F/P according to the following formula.

$F/P = 2.87 \times A_{495}/A_{280} - 0.35 \times A_{495}$，其中 A_{495}、A_{280} 分别代表 495 nm、280 nm 下的光吸收值,适当的 F/P 值应在 2～4。

$F/P = 2.87 \times A_{495}/A_{280} - 0.35 \times A_{495}$，$A_{495}$ and A_{280} represent the light absorption values at 495 nm and 280 nm respectively，and the appropriate F/P value should between 2 and 4.

6) 分装,4℃避光保存备用。

Aliquot fluorescein-labeled antibodies，and store at 4℃，shielded from light.

(3) 附录 Appendix：配制 pH 9.0～9.5 的碳酸盐缓冲液：Na_2CO_3 4.3 g、$NaHCO_3$ 8.6 g 溶入终体积为 500 ml 的超纯水中。

Dissolve 4.3 g Na_2CO_3 and 8.6 g $NaHCO_3$ in ultra-purified water at a final volume of 500 ml.

2. 四乙基罗丹明标记抗体的制备 Preparation of RB200 labeled antibodies

(1) 仪器与试剂 Required equipment and reagents：透析袋、Sephadex G50 柱、四乙基罗丹明(RB200)、无水丙醇、生理盐水和碳酸盐缓冲液(pH 9.0～9.5)。

Dialysis bag，Sephadex G25 column，RB200，anhydrous propanol，physiological saline，carbonate buffer (pH 9.0 to 9.5).

(2) 操作步骤 Protocol

1) 称取 1 g RB200 和 2 g 五氯化磷于研钵中仔细研磨 5 min,加入 10 ml 无水乙醇不断搅拌 5 min,再用滤纸过滤上述溶液,所得滤液将被用于抗体标记(注：RB200 可在五氯化磷的作用下转变成磺酰氯 SO_2Cl,后者在碱性条件下可与蛋白质的 ε-氨基结合,从而实现对抗体的标记)。

Place 1 g RB200 and 2 g phosphorus pentachloride in a mortar and grind carefully for 5 min，10 ml absolute ethanol are then added to the mortar and the mixture stirred for 5 min，The solution is then filtered through filter paper，and the filtrate retained for antibody labeling.

2) 取抗体(浓度一般在 20 mg/ml 左右)适量,按照每毫升抗体各加入 1 ml 生理盐水和碳酸盐缓冲液的比例稀释,然后逐滴加入 0.1 ml RB200 溶液,边加边搅拌。

Dilute the appropriate amount of antibody (generally about 20 mg/ml) according at a ratio of 1 ml normal saline and 1 ml of carbonate buffer. Add 0.1 ml RB200 solution to this solution drop by drop，under constant stirring.

3) 0～4℃结合 12～18 h,再用生理盐水透析 5～7 h。

Incubate at 0 to 4℃ for 12 to 18 hours to allow labeling of the antibodies，then dialyze the solution against normal saline for 5 to 7 hours.

4）经 Sephadex G50 柱层析，除去游离荧光素。

Use Sephadex G25 column to eliminate free RB200，as described above for fluorescein-5-isothiocyanate labeling

5）分装，4℃避光保存备用。

Aliquot fluorescein-labeled antibodies，and store at 4℃，shielded from light.

3. 藻红蛋白标记抗体的制备　Preparation of PE labeled antibodies

（1）仪器与试剂 Required equipment and reagents：Sephadex G25 柱、Sephacryl S-300 柱、纯化过的抗体（2.5 mg/ml）、纯化过的藻红蛋白（phycoerthrin，PE）、异双功能试剂（1.3 mg/ml SPDP 和 1.7 mg/ml SMCC）、77 mg/ml 二硫苏糖醇（DTT）、0.1 mmol N-乙基顺丁烯二酰亚胺（N-ethymaleimide，NEM）、PBS（不含 Ca^{2+}、Mg^{2+}）、甲醇、DMSO。

Sephadex G25 columns，Sephacryl S-300 columns，2.5 mg/ml purified antibodies，purified PE 1.3 mg/ml SPDP（3-(2-pyridyldithio) propionic acid N-hydroxysuccinimide ester），1.7 mg/ml SMCC（succinimidyltrans-4-(N-maleimidylmethy) cyclohexane-1-carboxlate），77 mg/ml dithiothreitol（DTT），0.1 mmol N-ethylmaleimide（NEM），PBS（Ca^{2+} and Mg^{2+} free），methanol，DMSO.

（2）操作步骤 Protocols

1）取 0.25 ml 保存在 60％$(NH)_4SO_4$ 中的 PE（4 mg/ml），经离心弃掉上清液，并用 0.25 ml PBS 重悬。

Centrifuge 0.25 ml phycoerthrin（PE）stored in 60％$(NH)_4SO_4$（4 mg/ml），discard the supernatant，and resuspend the pellet in 0.25 ml PBS.

2）将上述重悬的 PE 溶液在室温下用 150 ml PBS 透析 30 min，期间换液 2 次。

Dialyze the resuspended PE solution against 150 ml PBS at room temperature for 30 minutes，changing the PBS twice during this time.

3）调整透析后的 PE 溶液浓度在 1.4 mg/ml（共约有 0.7 ml 体积），加入 16 μl SPDP，室温孵育 2～3 h。

Adjust the concentration of the dialyzed PE solution to 1.4 mg/ml（final volume about 0.7 ml），add 16 μl SPDP，and store at room temperature for 2 to 3 hours.

4）取纯化的抗体 1 ml（2.5 mg/ml），加入 20 μl SMCC 溶液，室温孵育 1 h，制备 SMCC-抗体交联物。

To prepare cross-linked SMCC-antibodies，add 20 μl SMCC solution to 1 ml purified-antibodies（2.5 mg/ml）and incubate at room temperature for 1 hour.

5）加入 30 μl DTT 溶液到第三步交联好的 SPDP-PE 中，室温孵育 30 min。

Add 30 μl DTT solution to the cross-linked SPDP-PE solution prepared in step 3 and incubate at room temperature for 30 minutes.

6）用 Sephadex G25 柱层析纯化 SPDP-PE 和 SMCC-抗体交联物。

Purify cross-linked SPDP-PE and SMCC-antibodies using Sephadex G25 columns.

7）将纯化后的 SPDP-PE 和 SMCC-抗体交联物混合，4℃振荡过夜。

Combine the purified SPDP-PE and SMCC-antibodies and shake overnight at 4℃.

8) 加入 80 μl 的 0.1 mmol N-乙基顺丁烯二酰亚胺室温振荡孵育 30 min,终止反应。

Add 80 μl 0.1 mmol N-ethyl maleimide, incubate at room temperature for 30 minutes with gentle rotation to terminate the reaction.

9) 利用 Sephacryl S-300 柱层析分离纯化 PE 标记的抗体,用 PBS 洗脱,收集第一个洗脱峰。

Use a Sephacryl S-300 column to isolate the PE-labeled antibodies, eluting with PBS and collecting the first elution peak.

10) 分装,4℃避光保存备用。

Aliquot and store at 4℃ with shielding from light.

4. 四甲基罗丹明异硫氰酸酯标记抗体的制备　Preparation of TRITC labeled antibodies

(1) 仪器与试剂 Required equipment and reagents:透析袋、Bio-Gel P-6 层析柱、湿盒、纯化过的抗体、TRITC、0.01 mol/L PBS(pH 8.0)、DMSO、pH 9.0～9.5 的碳酸盐缓冲液(同前)。

Dialysis bag, Bio-Gel P-6 column, humidified chamber, purified antibodies, TRITC, 0.01 mol/L PBS (pH 8.0), DMSO, carbonate buffer (pH 9.0 to 9.5).

(2) 操作步骤 Protocols

1) 取 10 ml 抗体(6 mg/ml)放入透析袋在 pH 9.0～9.5 的碳酸盐缓冲液中透析过夜,将透析后的抗体转移至一小塑料管中。

Centrifuge 10 ml antibodies (6 mg/ml) and transfer to a dialysis bag, dialysis overnight in carbonate buffer of pH 9.0 to 9.5, then transfer the dialyzed-antibodies to a small plastic tube.

2) 称取 TRITC 1 mg,用 DMSO 溶解制成浓度为 1 mg/ml 的溶液。

Centrifuge 1 mg TRITC powder and dissolve in DMSO at a final concentration of 1 mg/ml.

3) 取上述 TRITC 溶液 300 μl 逐滴加入到透析过的抗体溶液中,室温下避光搅拌 2 h。

Add 300 μl of the above solution slowly to the dialyzed-antibodies and gently stir for 2 hours at room temperature.

4) Bio-Gel P-6 层析柱,用 PBS 洗脱,收集先流出的红色结合物。

Load the above solution onto a Bio-Gel P-6 column, elute with PBS and collect the first eluent fraction containing the TRITC-antibody conjugates.

5) 分装,4℃避光保存备用。

Aliquot and store at 4℃, with shielding from light.

(二) 免疫荧光染色　Immunofluorescence staining

1. 直接法　Direct staining

(1) 染色:给经过固定的细胞或组织材料滴加稀释至染色效价的荧光标记抗体,在室温或 37℃孵育 30 min。染色的整个过程,切片应放置在湿盒中并避光。

Dilute the fluorescent labeled antibodies to an appropriate potency and drip solution onto cells or tissues immobilized on glass slides. Incubate at room temperature at 37℃ for

30 minutes inside a humidified chamber.

（2）洗片：弃掉存留的荧光抗体，然后用 pH 7.2 或 pH 7.4 的 0.01 mol/L PBS 洗涤切片 2 次，每次 5 min，最后再用纯水洗去结晶盐。

Tip the slides to remove solution containing the fluorescent antibodies, then immerse the slides twice in 0.01 mol/L PBS (pH 7.2 or 7.4) for 5 minutes. Finally, gently rinse the slides with purified water to remove crystalline salts

（3）用 50% 缓冲(0.5 mol/L 的磷酸盐缓冲液，pH 9.0～9.5)甘油封固玻片，镜检。

Seal the samples with a drop of 50% buffered glycerol (0.5 mol/L PBS, pH 9.0 to 9.5) and coverslip and examine under a light microscope.

2. 间接法 Indirect staining

常用的间接法主要有两种：双层法和夹心法。

Two methods in common use：double staining and sandwich staining.

（1）双层法 Double staining

1）在固定的组织或细胞切(涂、爬)片上加特定比例的一抗，置于染色用的湿盒中 37℃ 孵育 30 min。

Add diluted, unlabeled primary antibodies on glass slides, incubate in a humidified chamber at 37℃ for 30 minutes.

2）用 pH 7.2 的 0.01 mol/L PBS 洗涤 2 次，每次 5 min，最后再用吸水纸吸去残留的液体。

Immerse the slides twice in 0.01 mol/L PBS (pH 7.2) for 5 minutes and absorb the residual liquid with absorbent paper.

3）滴加荧光标记的二抗，置于湿盒中 37℃ 孵育 30 min，再用 PBS 洗涤 2 次，每次 5 min，用吸水纸吸去残留的液体。

Drip fluorescently labeled secondary antibodies that specifically bind to the unlabeled primary antibodies onto the slides and incubate in a humidified chamber at 37℃ for 30 minutes. Wash slides twice with 0.01 mol/L PBS for 5 minutes and absorb the residual liquid with absorbent paper.

4）缓冲甘油封片，显微镜下观察。

Seal the slides with 50% buffered glycerol, and examine under a light microscope.

（2）夹心法 Sandwich staining：夹心法是一种用未标记的抗原检测组织或细胞中抗体的方法。

Sandwich staining is a method for detecting antibodies in tissues or cells with unmarked antigens.

1）在固定的组织细胞切(涂)片上滴加一定比例的特异性抗原，置于染色用的湿盒中 37℃ 孵育 30 min。

Drop diluted, specific antigen onto glass slides, incubate in a humidified chamber at 37℃ for 30 minutes.

2）用 pH 7.2 的 0.01 mol/L PBS 洗涤 2 次，每次 5 min，最后再用吸水纸吸去残留的液体。

Wash the slides twice with 0.01 mol/L PBS (pH 7.2) for 5 minutes and absorb the residual liquid with absorbent paper.

3) 滴加可与抗原结合的特异性荧光标记抗体，置于湿盒中 37℃ 孵育 30 min。

Cover samples with one-to-several drops of fluorescently labelled antibodies that specifically bind the target antigen and incubate in a humidified chamber at 37℃ for 30 minutes.

4) 用 pH 7.2 的 0.01 mol/L PBS 洗涤 2 次，每次 5 min，最后再用吸水纸吸去残留的液体。

Immerse the slides twice in 0.01 mol/L PBS (pH 7.2) for 5 minutes and absorb the residual liquid with absorbent paper.

5) 缓冲甘油封片，显微镜下观察。

Seal the slides with 50% buffered glycerol, and examine under a light microscope.

（三）免疫荧光染色的检测　Detection of immunofluorescence staining

免疫荧光标记的组织或细胞玻片可用荧光显微镜、激光扫描共聚焦显微镜等进行检测。

Immunofluorescent labeled tissues and cells on glass slides can be detected by fluorescence microscopy or laser scanning confocal microscopy.

四、免疫酶技术　Immunoenzymatic assay

免疫酶技术，借助于酶细胞化学反应而非荧光标记来检测抗原的存在。主要有酶标抗体法和非标记抗体酶法两种主要形式。

Immunoenzymatic assay detects the presence of antigens based on *in situ* enzymatic reactions. There are two primary techniques used are: enzyme-labeled antibody methods and non-labeled antibody enzyme methods.

（一）酶标抗体法　Enzyme-labeled antibody methods

1. 酶标抗体的制备　Preparation of enzyme-labeled antibodies

可用于抗体标记的酶一般应具有以下几点：①酶催化的底物必须是特异性的，容易被显示，易于在光学显微镜下或电子显微镜下观察；②用于免疫化学的酶要易于获得，便于商品化和标准化；③在中性 pH 值时，酶应比较稳定，标记在抗体上的酶应在 1~2 年内活性不变；④所形成的终产物沉淀必须稳定，不能从酶活性部位向周围组织弥散，而影响组织学定位；⑤酶与抗体的连接不能影响抗体的活性；⑥在被检测的细胞或组织中，不能存在与标记酶相同的内源性酶或作用相似的酶。常用的标记酶有辣根过氧化物酶（horseradish peroxidase，HRP）、碱性磷酸酶（alkaline phosphatase，ALP）、葡萄糖氧化酶（glucose oxidase，GOD）等。

Enzymes that can be used to label antibodies should generally have the following characteristics: ①Enzyme-catalyzed substrates must be specific and easy to display, and easy to observe under light or electron microscopy. ②Enzymes for immunochemistry should be readily available, commercialized and standardized. ③At neutral pH, the enzymes should be relatively stable，and the activity of the enzymes linked to the antibodies should remain unchanged for 1 to 2 years．④ The precipitated enzymatic end-products should be stable and not diffuse from the site of enzyme activity to surrounding tissues，which would adversely affect histological localization．⑤The linkage of the enzyme to the antibody should not affect the binding specificity or activity of the antibody．⑥Endogenous enzymes or enzymes with similar functions should not be expressed in the target cells or tissues．Enzymes commonly used as antibody markers include：horseradish peroxidase (HRP)，alkaline phosphatase (ALP)，and glucose oxidase (GOD)．

　　酶标抗体的制备与荧光素标记抗体的制备不同，它需借助偶联剂将酶连接到抗体分子上。常用的偶联剂有戊二醛、过碘酸钠、马来酰亚胺等。这些偶联剂通过共价键与抗体形成不可逆的结合，且不影响酶和抗体的活性，不会导致酶标抗体与细胞组织的其他成分发生非特异性结合。

The preparation of enzyme-labeled antibodies is different from the fluorescein-labeled antibodies．Commonly used coupling agents for linking enzymes to antibodies include：glutaraldehyde，sodium periodate and maleimide．The binding of these coupling agents to enzymes and antibodies is irreversible，since covalent bonds are formed．It is essential that the coupling agent does not inhibit the activities of the enzymes or antibodies or cause non-specific binding of enzyme-labeled antibodies to components of cells or tissues．

　　2. 染色方法　Staining methods

　　酶标抗体的染色同样包括直接法和间接法两种，以间接法为主。间接法主要包括以下步骤。

Staining cells and tissues with enzyme-labeled antibodies can be accomplished using both direct and indirect methods．Indirect staining involves the following steps.

　　(1) 细胞组织切(涂、爬)片的准备与固定。

Preparation and fixation of cell or tissue sections.

　　(2) 用 PBS 或其他缓冲液洗涤切片 3 次，每次 2 min。冷冻切片洗涤后进入第三步；而石蜡切片在洗涤后直接进行第四步。注意当用 ALP 标记的抗体时，应禁用二甲胂酸钠缓冲液洗涤，因为后者可使 ALP 失活。

Wash the sections three times with PBS or other buffer for 2 minutes each time to dissolve and remove the OCT embedding agent from the frozen section．However，when using ALP-labeled antibodies，washing with sodium dimethylarsenate buffer should be avoided because the latter can inactivate ALP．Wash the paraffin sections and proceed directly to the fourth step．

　　(3) 根据需要，用 0.3% 过氧化氢处理切片 15～30 min，封闭内源性氧化酶的作用。PBS 洗涤 2 次，每次 2 min(应用 ALP 标记的抗体时可省略此过程)。

Treat sections with 0.3% hydrogen peroxide for 15 to 30 minutes to block the effect of endogenous oxidase．Wash with PBS twice，2 minutes each time (Omit this process when using ALP-labeled antibodies)．

（4）在室温条件下，将切片放入含 0.05%Tween-20 的 PBS 中处理 5 min，以增强组织的通透性。

Immerse sections in the PBS containing 0.05% Tween-20 at room temperature for 5 minutes to enhance tissue permeability.

（5）用 4% 的 block ace 或 0.01%~1% 的 BSA 在湿盒中孵育切片 15~25 min，以阻断抗体与组织的非特应性结合。

Incubate sections in a humidified chamber with 4% block ace or 0.01% to 1% BSA for 15 to 25 minutes to block the nonspecific binding of antibodies to tissues.

（6）轻轻弃掉上述孵育液，根据需要滴加含 0.2%BSA、0.05% NaN$_3$ 的经 PBS 稀释的一抗。通常，每片滴加 50~80 μl，室温下湿盒中孵育 1~2 h，免疫电子显微镜标本需要在 4℃ 下过夜。注意此处漂洗时应与对照组分开洗涤以防发生交叉污染。

Gently discard the incubation solution and add the PBS-diluted primary antibodies containing 0.2% BSA and 0.05% NaN$_3$. Usually, each section dropping 50 to 80 μl antibody, incubate in a humidified chamber at room temperature for 1 to 2 hours. Immune electron microscopic specimens need to be stored overnight at 4℃ (Note: The rinse should be separated from the control group to prevent cross-contamination.)

（7）PBS 洗涤 3 次，每次 2 min，以除去非特异性结合的抗体。

Wash sections with PBS three times, 2 minutes each time, to remove non-specifically bond or adsorbed antibodies.

（8）用含 0.05%Tween-20 的 PBS 洗涤 2 min 后，滴加由 PBS（含 0.2%BSA、1%血清）稀释的 HRP 酶标二抗，室温下湿盒内孵育 45~60 min。

Wash with PBS buffer (containing 0.05% Tween-20) for 2 minutes. Cover samples with one-to-several drops of HRP labeled secondary antibodies diluted to an appropriate concentration with PBS (containing 0.2% BSA, 1% normal serum) and incubate in a humidified chamber at room temperature for 45 to 60 minutes.

（9）PBS 洗涤 3 次，每次 2 min。

Wash sections with PBS three times, 2 minutes each time.

（10）显色：HRP 标记抗体的显色剂为含有 0.01%~0.1% H$_2$O$_2$、0.01%~0.05% DAB、0.01~0.1 mol/L Tris-HCl(pH7.4) 的缓冲液。切片经 PBS 漂洗后，在室温条件下置入上述显色液中显色，镜检控制显色时间与速度。

Coloring: The chromogenic agent of HRP labeled antibody is the buffer which containing 0.01% to 0.1% H$_2$O$_2$, 0.01% to 0.05% 3,3'-diaminobenzidine (DAB), 0.01 to 0.1 mol/L Tris-HCl (pH 7.4). Rinse sections with PBS, and color in the above chromogenic agent at room temperature. Observe under a microscope to monitor the time and speed of color development.

（11）流水或 PBS 终止显色。

Wash in running water or PBS to terminate coloring.

（12）系列乙醇脱水、Hemo-De 透明、DPX 封固、镜检。

Ethanol gradient dehydration，Hemo-De transparency，DPX sealing, and microscopic examination.

（二）非标记抗体酶法　Non-labeled antibody enzyme method

非标记抗体酶法由 Sternberger 等在酶标法的基础上发展而成，能有效降低背景，能最大程度保留抗体的活性，灵敏度高。主要有酶桥法（enzyme bridge method）和过氧化物酶抗过氧化物酶法（peroxidase antiperoxidase method，PAP method），又以后者的应用较为广泛。

Non-labeled antibody methods include enzyme bridging methods, where a second non-labeled antibody is used as a molecular bridge between the primary antibody and a third antibody that binds a reporter enzyme used for detection. High specificity and low background staining in these assays are the result of the use of bridging antibodies that specifically bind to the Fc domain of both the primary and tertiary antibodies. Among several variations of this assay the peroxidase antiperoxidase (PAP) method is widely used.

这两种方法均需先用酶免疫动物，制备效价高、特异性强的抗酶抗体，然后在第二抗体（亦称桥抗体）的作用下，将抗酶抗体与和组织抗原结合在一起的第一抗体连接起来，进而再将酶结合在抗酶抗体上，最后经呈色反应来显示抗原的分布。所不同的是，在 PAP 法中，通常先让抗酶抗体与酶形成复合物（如 PAP 复合物），然后在桥抗体的帮助下，一次性将抗酶抗体、酶与一抗结合。

Enzyme bridging assays require：① primary antibodies that specifically bind a target antigen in cells or tissues；② a bridging enzyme that binds the Fc domain of both the primary antibodies and tertiary antibodies；③ polyclonal tertiary antibodies that bind to distinct antigenic sites on the surface of reporter enzymes，without inhibiting their enzymatic activities. The ability of the tertiary antibody to bind distinct sites on the reporter enzymes，allows the formation of antibody/enzyme complexes that significantly amplify the production of the colored product of the enzymatic reaction, thereby increasing the signal for antigen detection. In the PAP assay，cells or tissues under investigation are first exposed to the primary antibodies for an extended period，washed to remove the unbound antibodies，and then exposed to the bridging antibodies. After washing to remove the unbound bridging antibodies，the samples are exposed to preformed complexes (PAP complexes) between tertiary antibodies and horseradish peroxidase (HRP). After a final washing，the samples are incubated with 3，3'-diaminobenzidine (DAB) and hydrogen peroxide (H_2O_2) to generate an insoluble colored enzymatic reaction product that marks the site of the target antigen.

在此过程中，任何抗体均未被酶标记，酶是通过免疫学原理与抗酶抗体结合，避免了共价连接对抗体和酶活性的损害，同时还提高了方法的敏感性，并节省第一抗体的用量。

In this method，none of the antibodies are covalently linked to reporter enzymes. Rather，reporter enzymes are indirectly linked to the primary antibodies via bridging antibodies that also bind tertiary antibody/detection enzyme complexes, which form via binding between various sites on surface of the reporter enzymes and the tertiary antibody

Fab antigen binding domains. Although complicated, enzyme bridging assays have several advantages compared to other direct enzyme binding methods, including the avoidance of potential damage to reporter enzymes or secondary antibodies caused by creating covalent bonds, improved sensitivity for antigen detection, and the ability to used low concentrations of primary antibodies.

1. PAP 复合物的制备 Preparation of PAP complex

(1) 试剂 Required reagents：1 mg/ml HRP 溶液、2 mg/ml HRP 溶液、生理盐水、0.1 mol/L HCl、1 mol/L HCl、0.1 mol/L NaOH、1 mol/L NaOH、饱和硫酸铵溶液、50% 硫酸铵溶液、透析液(48.6 g NaCl，1.5 mol/L NaOOCCH$_3$ 30 ml，1.5 mol/L (NH$_4$)$_2$SO$_4$ 30 ml，超纯水 5.94 L)。

1 mg/ml HRP solution, 2 mg/ml HRP solution, normal saline, 0.1 mol/L HCl, 1 mol/L HCl, 0.1 mol/L NaOH, 1 mol/L NaOH, saturated ammonium sulfate solution, 50% ammonium sulfate solution, dialysate buffer [48.6 g NaCl, 1.5 mol/L NaOOCCH$_3$ 30 ml, 1.5 mol/L (NH$_4$)$_2$SO$_4$ 30 ml, ultrapure water 5.94 L].

(2) 步骤 Protocols

1) 按常规免疫学方法制备抗 HRP 血清。

Prepare anti-HRP serum by routine immunological method.

2) 取 10.5 ml 抗 HRP 血清，加 7.6 ml HRP 溶液(1 mg/ml)，混匀后，室温放置 1 h。

Mix 10.5 ml anti-HRP serum with 7.6 ml HRP solution (1 mg/ml) at room temperature for 1 hour.

3) 4℃，16 000×g 离心 15 min，小心弃掉上清液。

Centrifuge at 4℃ for 15 min at 16 000×g and discard the supernatant carefully.

4) 用预冷的生理盐水溶解沉淀物，4℃，16 000×g 离心 15 min，重复 4 次。

Dissolve pellet with precooled normal saline, centrifuge at 4℃ for 15 min at 16 000×g, and repeat four times.

5) 加入 15.3 ml HRP 溶液(2 mg/ml)，室温持续搅拌 1 h。

Add 15.3 ml HRP solution (2 mg/ml), stirring at room temperature for 1 hour.

6) 用 1 mol/L HCl 和 0.1 mol/L HCl 调 pH 值至 2.3。沉淀物全部溶解变清时，立即用 1 mol/L NaOH 和 0.1 mol/L NaOH 调 pH 值至 7.2。

Adjust the pH to 2.3 with 1 mol/L HCl and 0.1 mol/L HCl, the pellet will dissolve and become clear, and immediately adjust the pH to 7.2 with 1 mol/L and 0.1 mol/L NaOH.

7) 慢慢加入等体积的饱和硫酸铵，0℃放置 45 min。

Add the same volume of saturated ammonium sulfate slowly and place at 0℃ for 45 minutes.

8) 0℃，35 000×g 离心 15 min，所得沉淀物用 50%硫酸铵洗涤 2 次。

Centrifuge at 0℃, 35 000×g for 15 minutes, wash the pellet twice with 50% ammonium sulfate.

9）用 10.5 ml 超纯水溶解沉淀物，置入透析袋中 4℃透析过夜。

Add 10. 5 ml ultrapure water to dissolve the pellet，transfer to dialysate bag and dialyze at 4℃ overnight.

10）4℃离心，收集上清液，加适量透析液使体积至 10.5 ml，分装后于 4℃保存。

Centrifuge at 4℃，collect the supernatant，add proper dialysate buffer to 10. 5 ml，aliquot and store at 4℃.

2. PAP 染色方法　PAP staining method

染色步骤包括：①切片准备及第一抗体孵育前处理，步骤同酶标抗体染色间接法的 1～5步；②切片与特异性一抗 4℃孵育 24 h；③用过量的桥抗体孵育；④用离体制得的 PAP 复合物（常用 1：30～300 稀释）室温下孵育 1～1.5 h，使其能够被桥抗体连接在第一抗体上；⑤用 DAB－H₂O₂ 溶液显色，镜下控制显色程度；⑥系列乙醇脱水，二甲苯透明，DPX 封固，镜检。

The staining steps include：①Section preparation and primary antibody pre-incubation are the same as the 1 to 5 steps of indirect enzyme-labeled antibody staining；②Incubate sections with specific primary antibodies at 4℃ for 24 hours；③ Incubate sections with excessive bridge-antibodies；④Incubate with prepared PAP complexes （usually diluted at 1：30 to 300）at room temperature for 1 to 1. 5 hours，to bind the primary antibodies via bridging-antibodies；⑤Stain with DAB－H₂O₂ and monitor the degree of color under a microscope；⑥ Proceed with ethanol gradient dehydration，xylene transparency，DPX sealing，and microscopic examination.

五、亲合组织化学　Affinity histochemistry

随着免疫组织化学方法的广泛应用，一些新的技术创新也不断涌现。其中最具代表性的就是一些具有双价或多价结合力的物质如植物凝集素（lectin）、生物素（biotin）和葡萄球菌 A 蛋白（staphylococcal protein A，SPA）等被应用于免疫细胞化学技术，从而建立了 SPA－HRP 法、ABC 法、BRAB 法和 LAB 法等一些新的细胞组织化学技术。这些技术一方面区别于古老的组织化学的分解、置换、氧化和还原，另一方面在本质上又不属于抗原抗体反应。因此，Bayer 在 1976 年将其命名为亲合组织化学（affinity histochemistry）。

Novel methods in immunohistochemistry have emerged in recent years，many based on the use bivalent or multivalent binding proteins and their ligands，such as：lectins/complex polysaccharides，staphylococcal protein A （SPA）/IgG，and avidin/biotin. Methods currently in wide use include：SPA－HRP，ABC，BRAB and LAB. Together，these methods their applications comprise a subfield of immunohistochemistry termed "affinity histochemistry" by Bayer in 1976.

目前，亲合组织化学包括植物凝集素与糖类、抗生物素与生物素、葡萄球菌 A 蛋白与 IgG、阳离子与阴离子、激素、维生素、糖及类脂质作用部位和受体等。由于抗原与抗体的相互作用从本质上讲也是一种亲和作用，所以，抗原抗体反应亦属于亲和组织化学范畴。亲合细胞化学（affinity cytochemistry）引入免疫细胞化学后使得免疫细胞化学的敏感性得到进一步提高,更有利于在细胞或亚细胞水平对微量抗原(或抗体)的定位进行研究。现以抗生物素-生物素免疫细胞化学染色为例,简要介绍亲和组织化学技术。

At present, affinity histochemistry-based methods incorporate diverse types of binding pairs, including plant-derived lectins and complex sugars, egg whites-derived avidin and biotin, staphylococcal bacteria-derived protein A and IgGs, and tissue-derived proteins and hormones/vitamins/lipids, etc. (for example, annexin-V and phosphtidylserine). Since the interaction of an antigen with an antibody is also based on mutual affinity, the antigen-antibody reaction can also be regarded as a topic in affinity histochemistry. The introduction of affinity-based techniques to immunohistochemistry has significantly increased the ability to detect and locate trace antigens at the tissue, cell and subcellular levels. The following is a brief introduction to affinity histochemistry techniques, taking avidin-biotin immunocytochemical staining as an example.

(一) 抗生物素-生物素免疫细胞化学染色的原理　Principle of avidin-biotin immunocytochemical staining

人们对抗生物素-生物素亲和作用的发现源于养殖实践。研究发现,来自饲料中鸡蛋白成分的抗生物素(又称卵白素,avidin)能和生物素(又称维生素 H)结合,从而导致"维生素 H 缺乏症"的发生。进一步研究发现,抗生物素与生物素的这种亲和力远比抗原与抗体间的亲和力要高出 100 万倍,且不会影响彼此的生物学活性。免疫细胞化学工作者受这一特殊现象的启发,便建立起抗生物素-生物素免疫细胞化学染色方法。

The discovery of high-affinity biotin binding proteins began with studies showing that inclusion of egg whites in animal feed can produce "vitamin H deficiency." Follow-up investigations revealed that egg whites contain a protein, avidin, which binds to "vitamin H" (biotin) with high affinity. Further studies determined that the affinity of avidin for biotin is more than 1 million times stronger than the binding affinity of antibodies for antigens. Based on these observations, immunologists have developed many novel biotin/avidin-based immunocytochemical staining methods.

(二) 抗生物素-生物素免疫细胞化学染色方法　Avidin-biotin immunocytochemical staining method

常见的抗生物素-生物素免疫细胞化学染色方法主要有抗生物素-生物素-过氧化物酶复合物技术(avidin biotin-peroxidase complex technique,ABC 法)、桥抗生物素-生物素技术(bridged avidin-biotin technique,BRAB 法)、标记生物素-抗生物素技术(labelled avidin-biotin technique,LAB 法)3 种,其中以抗生物素-生物素-过氧化物酶复合物技术最为常用。

Common avidin-biotin immunocytochemical staining techniques include the: avidin biotin-peroxidase complex (ABC), bridged avidin-biotin (BRAB), and labeled avidin-biotin (LAB) methods. Among these, the ABC method is the most often used.

1. 抗生物素-生物素-过氧化物酶复合物(ABC)技术的原理　Principle of avidin-biotin-peroxidase complex technology (ABC)

ABC 法利用抗生物素分别将生物素标记的二抗和生物素标记的酶连接起来。与 LAB

法和 BRAB 法不同之处在于：①一抗不被标记物所标记；②生物素标记的二抗与 ABC 相连接；③ABC 是通过先将过氧化酶结合在生物素上、再将生物素-过氧化物酶连接物与过量的抗生物素蛋白反应而制备的。ABC 法具有特异性强、敏感度高、背景染色浅等优点。

This method uses unlabeled primary antibodies, biotin-labeled secondary antibodies, biotin-labeled reporter enzymes and avidin. Three layers of molecules are formed on cells or tissues stained using this method：① primary antibodies bound to the target antigen via their Fab domains. ② secondary antibodies bound to the Fc domains of the primary antibodies via their Fab domains. ③ ABC bound to the secondary antibodies via biotin covalently bound to the Fc domain of the secondary antibodies. ABC containing multiple reporter enzymes are prepared by mixing biotin-labeled peroxidase molecules with avidin, which binds biotin at multiple high-affinity binding sites. By contrast to the ABC method, the BRAB and LAB methods require biotin-labels primary antibodies.

2. 试剂　Required reagents

特异性抗体（单克隆或多克隆）、生物素标记的二抗、ABC、丙酮、0.01 mol/L PBS（pH 7.2~7.6）、DAB-H_2O_2 液、0.05 mol/L Tris-HCl 液（pH7.6）、抗体稀释液、DPX 封固液。

Specific antibodies（monoclonal or polyclonal），biotinylated secondary antibodies, ABC；acetone, 0.01 mol/L PBS（pH 7.2~7.6），DAB-H_2O_2 solution, 0.05 mol/L Tris-HCl solution（pH 7.6），antibody dilution buffer，DPX mountant.

3. 操作步骤　Protocols

（1）切片的处理：石蜡切片需先经脱蜡，然后用系列乙醇脱水；细胞涂（爬）片用含丙酮的甲醛（福尔马林）固定液固定 30 s；冷冻切片可用丙酮固定 10 min 左右。0.01 mol/L PBS 洗涤 3 次，每次 5 min。

Slice processing：Dewax paraffin sections first, then dehydrate with a series of ethanol. Fix cell smears（slides）with acetone-containing formalin fixative for 30 seconds, fix frozen sections with acetone for 10 minutes. Wash with 0.01 mol/L PBS 5 minutes for three times.

（2）加入一抗，室温孵育 15 min 或 4℃孵育 24 h。

Add the first antibodies，incubate for 15 minutes at room temperature or incubate for 24 hours at 4℃.

（3）用 PBS 洗涤 3 次，每次 5 min。

Wash sections with PBS three times，5 minutes each time.

（4）加生物素标记的第二抗体，室温孵育 2 h。

Add biotinylated secondary antibodies and incubate for 2 hours at room temperature.

（5）用 PBS 洗涤 3 次，每次 5 min。

Wash sections with PBS three times，5 minutes each time.

（6）加 ABC 置室温作用 30 min。

Add the ABC at room temperature for 30 minutes.

（7）用 PBS 洗涤 3 次，每次 5 min。

Wash sections with PBS three times，5 minutes each time.

（8）用 DAB－H_2O_2 液显色，镜下控制显色程度。

Color sections with DAB－H_2O_2 solution，control the degree of coloration under the microscope.

（9）苏木素复染。

Counterstain with hematoxylin.

（10）系列乙醇脱水，二甲苯透明，DPX 封固，镜检。

Series ethanol dehydration， xylene transparent， DPX sealing， microscopic examination.

4. 注意事项　Notes

一般实验过程中，当生物素与抗生物素的摩尔浓度之比为 1∶4 时，能获得最佳满意效果，宜在应用前 30 min 用 0.05 mol/L 的 Tris－HCl 液(pH7.6)进行配制。

Experience has shown that when the molar ratio of biotin to avidin is 1∶4，the best satisfactory results are obtained，it should be prepared with 0.05 mol/L Tris－HCl solution (pH 7.6)30 minutes before application.

5. 附录　Appendix

（1）抗体稀释液配置：0.1％ BSA、0.02％ KH_2PO_4、0.29％ Na_2HPO_4 • $12H_2O$、0.8％ NaCl、0.02％ KCl、0.05％ Tween－20 溶液。

Antibody dilution buffer containing 0.1％ BSA，0.02％ KH_2PO_4，0.29％ Na_2HPO_4 • $12H_2O$，0.8％ NaCl，0.02％ KCl，0.05％ Tween－20 solution.

（2）DPX 封固液配置：distren 10 g、5 ml 酸二丁、35 ml 二甲苯。

DPX mountant containing distren 10 g，5 ml dibutyl acid and 3 ml xylene.

第三节 ◉ 免疫沉淀与免疫共沉淀
Immunoprecipitation and co-immunoprecipitation

一、基本概念　Basic concepts

免疫沉淀(immunoprecipitation)是利用抗体可与抗原特异性结合的特性，将抗原(常为靶蛋白)从混合体系沉淀下来，初步分离靶蛋白的一种方法。

Immunoprecipitation is a method for isolating or concentrating a target antigen (often a target protein) from tissue or cellular extracts, based on the specific binding of antibodies to the antigen.

免疫共沉淀(co-immunoprecipitation)是一种在体外探测两个蛋白分子间是否存在特异性相互作用的一种方法。其原理是如果两个蛋白在体外体系能够发生特异性相互作用的话，那么当用一种蛋白的抗体进行免疫沉淀时，另一个蛋白也会被同时沉淀下来。与酵母双杂交技术不同的是，免疫共沉淀技术所利用的是抗原和抗体间的免疫反应，是一种在体外非细胞环境中研究蛋白质与蛋白质相互作用的方法。

Co-immunoprecipitation is a method of detecting binding between two or more proteins in tissue or cellular extracts. Co-immunoprecipitation of proteins in *in vitro* systems is often taken as evidence for binding or interactions between the proteins *in vivo*. Typically, immunoprecipitation is carried out using antibodies that bind to a single target protein, and addition antibodies are used to detect co-precipitated proteins.

不难看出,免疫共沉淀与免疫沉淀技术所使用的原理与方法大致相似,所不同的是,在免疫共沉淀中,对靶蛋白的结合与沉淀由另一个与之发生相互作用的蛋白替代。在免疫共沉淀或免疫沉淀的基础上,通过进一步与其他技术结合,如聚丙烯酰胺凝胶电泳,还可对靶蛋白的分子量等特性进行鉴定。

The principles and methods used in immunoprecipitation and co-immunoprecipitation techniques are similar. The molecular weights and identities of co-immunoprecipitated proteins can be determined using techniques, such as polyacrylamide gel electrophoresis and Western blot analysis. A useful control in these experiments is to repeat the immunoprecipitation using antibodies that recognize one or more of the co-immunoprecipitated proteins in the original experiment.

二、抗体的选择 Selection of antibodies

(一)多克隆抗体 Polyclonal antibodies

多克隆抗体因其制备相对简单,可与靶蛋白分子的多个位点结合,所形成的抗原抗体复合物较稳定因而应用的最为广泛。但多克隆抗体的缺点在于非特异性结合较多,常会导致反应本底升高和一定的假阳性结果。

Polyclonal antibodies are often used for immunoprecipitation because they comprise a mixture of antibodies that often bind to several different sites on a protein or different configurations of short peptide components of the protein. The ability to bind multiple sites or peptide configurations is important since successful immunoprecipitation depends upon the ability of the antibodies to bind to the target protein in its native configuration. A disadvantage of polyclonal antibodies is that they sometimes display non-specific binding, which can increase the immunoprecipitation background noise and in certain cases produce false positive results.

(二)单克隆抗体 Monoclonal antibodies

与多克隆抗体相比,单克隆抗体往往只结合一种抗原表位,具有单一结合的特异性,所以发生非特异结合的机会少,可被用于确定靶蛋白上某一部位的特殊结构,甚至可被用于区分相同靶蛋白的不同形式如构象变化和修饰。但反过来,单克隆抗体仅与单一表位结合的特性也会引起具有同一表位的不同靶蛋白间的交叉反应。

Compared with polyclonal antibodies, monoclonal antibodies usually bind only a single antigenic site or peptide configuration, and therefore produce less non-specific binding. Based on the considerations mentioned above, however, it is essential to prescreen monoclonal antibodies for the ability to immunoprecipitate the target protein in its native configuration before preceding to large-scale immunoprecipitation experiments. Occasionally, monoclonal antibodies can produce confusing results if they bind epitopes that are present on more than one protein.

三、免疫沉淀方法　Immunoprecipitation

免疫沉淀的靶蛋白一般来自细胞裂解液,可以是被同位素标记的也可以是未被标记的。若为前者,免疫沉淀后再经聚丙烯酰胺凝胶电泳,只需压片即可检测到靶蛋白的存在;若为后者,经免疫沉淀和聚丙烯酰凝胶电泳后,尚需借助银染或免疫印迹进行鉴定。

Immunoprecipitated target proteins are typically derived from cell lysates and may be isotopically labeled or unlabeled. If the former, after immunoprecipitation and then by polyacrylamide gel electrophoresis, only the tablet can detect the presence of the target protein; if the latter, after immunoprecipitation and polyacrylamide gel electrophoresis, it is still necessary to use silver dyeing or immunoblotting for identification.

(一)所需试剂　Required reagents

改良的 RIPA 缓冲液、PBS、TSA 缓冲液、0.05 mol/L Tris 缓冲液(pH 6.8)、2× SDS 蛋白上样缓冲液、抗体、sepharose、蛋白 A、蛋白 G。

Modified Radioimmunoprecipitation (RIPA) buffer, PBS, TSA buffer, 0.05 mol/L Tris buffer (pH6.8), 2× SDS protein loading buffer, antibodies, Sepharose, Protein A, Protein G.

(二)方法　Protocols

(1)用冰冷的 PBS 洗涤贴壁细胞 2 次,弃干净 PBS。对于悬浮细胞则用台式离心机以 800～1 000 r/min 转速通过离心洗涤。

Wash adherent cells twice with ice-cold PBS, and discard the PBS (For suspension cells, give them PBS wash and centrifuge at 800 to 1 000 r/min).

(2)给细胞培养瓶中加入冰冷的改良 RIPA 缓冲液。RIPA 缓冲液的用量按照 1 ml 每 10^7 个细胞/100 mm 培养面/150 cm^2 瓶或 0.5 ml 每 $5×10^6$ 细胞/60 mm 培养面/75 cm^2 瓶计算。

Add ice-cold modified RIPA buffer (1 ml per 10^7 cells/100 mm dish/150 cm^2 flask; 0.5 ml per $5×10^6$ cells/60 mm dish/75 cm^2 flask) to the culture flask.

(3)用经蒸馏水预冷的橡皮或塑料细胞刮棒将贴壁细胞转移至离心管中,轻轻混匀细胞悬液,用振荡器在 4℃振荡 15 min 以裂解细胞。

Transfer adherent cells to a centrifuge tube with a rubber or plastic cell scraper precooled with purified water, mix the cell suspension gently, lyse cells by a shaker at 4℃ for 15 minutes.

(4)于 4℃,14 000×g 离心裂解液 15 min,迅速转移上清液至另一离心管中,弃掉沉淀物。

Centrifuge the lysate at 14 000 × g at 4℃ for 15 minutes, quickly transfer the supernatant to another centrifuge tube, and discard the pellet.

（5）准备蛋白 A(蛋白 G 或 sepharose)：用 PBS 洗涤蛋白 A(蛋白 G 或 sepharose)珠子 2 次，并将其用 PBS 调制成 50% 的悬液。

Prepare protein A (protein G or sepharose)：Wash protein A (protein G or sepharose) beads with PBS twice and restore to a 50% slurry with fresh PBS.

（6）每 1 ml 细胞裂解液上清液加入 100 μl 蛋白 A(蛋白 G 或 sepharose)，4℃，振荡 10 min，进行预清除。

Add 100 μl of protein A (protein G or sepharose) to 1 ml supernatant at 4℃, and shake for 10 minutes for pre-clearing.

（7）4℃，14 000×g 离心 10 min 移去蛋白 A(蛋白 G 或 sepharose)，转移上清液至一新离心管中。

Centrifuge at 14 000×g at 4℃ for 10 minutes, transfer the supernatant (protein) to a new centrifuge tube.

（8）用 Bradford 法(考马斯亮蓝染色法)测定蛋白浓度。应至少将细胞裂解液作 1∶10 稀释后再测定，这是因为存在于裂解液中的去污剂成分会干扰考马斯亮蓝的作用。

Determine protein concentration by using the Bradford method (Coomassie brilliant blue stain). (The cell lysate should be diluted at least 1∶10 before determination because the detergent component present in the lysate interferes with the effect of Coomassie brilliant blue).

（9）根据所测得的细胞裂解液蛋白浓度，用 PBS 将其稀释至 1 mg/ml 以降低缓冲体系中去污剂的浓度。但对于那些在细胞中表达水平较低的蛋白而言，10 mg/ml 这样更高的浓度可能对免疫沉淀更有效一些。

Dilute protein to 1 mg/ml with PBS to reduce the concentration of detergent in the buffer system (but for those proteins with lower expression levels in cells, higher concentration of 10 mg/ml may be more effective for immunoprecipitation).

（10）加入推荐体积的免疫沉淀抗体至 500 μl 细胞裂解液中。抗体的最适用量要根据每一细胞模型中免疫沉淀靶蛋白的数量来确定。

Add the recommended volume of immunoprecipitated antibodies to 500 μl cell lysate.

（11）将细胞裂解液与抗体轻轻混匀后孵育 2 h，或置摇床上振荡 4℃过夜。加入 100 μl 蛋白 A(蛋白 G 或 sepharose)轻轻振荡 1 h 或 4℃过夜以捕获免疫沉淀复合物。在多数情况下，加入 2 μg 兔抗小鼠 IgG 的桥连抗体可以增强对免疫复合物的捕获能力，这对于小鼠 IgG1 或由鸡所产生的低亲和力抗体尤为重要。

Gently mix the cell lysate with the antibodies and incubate for 2 hours, or shake on a shaker overnight at 4℃. Add 100 μl Protein A, gently shake for 1 hour or overnight at 4℃ to capture the immunoprecipitated complex (In most cases, the addition of 2 μg of bridging antibodies such as rabbit anti-mouse IgG enhances the ability to capture immune complexes, which is especially important for mouse IgG1 and low-affinity antibodies from chickens).

（12）通过脉冲离心（14 000 r/min，5 s）收集琼脂糖/sepharose 珠子，弃掉上清液，用

800 μl 冰冷的改良 RIPA 缓冲液洗涤珠子 3 次。

Collect the agarose/sepharose beads by pulse spins (14 000 r/min, 5 s), discard the supernatant, wash three times with 800 μl of ice-cold modified RIPA buffer.

（13）将琼脂糖/sepharose 珠子重悬于 60 μl 2× SDS 蛋白上样缓冲液中，轻轻混匀后煮沸 5 min，200×g 离心 1 min 弃掉珠子。

Resuspend agarose/sepharose beads in 60 μl 2× SDS protein loading buffer, lightly mix and boil for 5 minutes, and centrifuge for 1 minute at 200×g to discard the pellet.

（14）将上清液转移至一新离心管中 -20℃ 冻存或进行 SDS-PAGE 电泳。

Transfer the supernatant to a new centrifuge tube, stored at -20℃ or for SDS-PAGE electrophoresis.

（三）附录　Appendix

改良的 RIPA 缓冲液的组成(100 ml 体系)：50 mmol/L Tris - HCl(pH 7. 4)、NP - 40：1%脱氧胆酸钠(0. 25%)、NaCl(150 mmol/L)、EDTA(1 mmol/L)、PMSF(1 mmol/L)、抑肽酶、亮肽酶素、抑肽素(各 1 μg/ml)、Na_3VO_4(1 mmol/L)、NaF(1 mmol/L)。

Modified RIPA buffer (100 ml)：Tris - HCl (50 mmol/L, pH 7. 4), NP - 40 (1%), sodium deoxycholate (0. 25%), NaCl (150 mmol/L), EDTA (1 mmol/L), PMSF (1 mmol/L), aprotinin (1 μg/ml), leupeptin (1 μg/ml), aprotinin (1 μg/ml), Na_3VO_4 (1 mmol/L), NaF (1 mmol/L).

第四节 ⊙ 免疫印迹
Immunoblotting

一、概述　Overview

免疫印迹(immunoblotting)又称蛋白质印迹(Western blotting)，是一种借助特异性抗体鉴定抗原的有效方法。该方法是在凝胶电泳和固相免疫测定技术基础上发展起来的一种免疫生化技术，既具有凝胶电泳的高分辨率，又具备固相免疫测定的高特异性和高灵敏性，可检测 1~5 ng 的中等大小蛋白。其优点是方法简便、标本可长期保存、结果便于比较，故被广泛应用于分子生物学等领域，成为一种常用的研究方法。

Immunoblotting, also known as Western blotting, is an effective method for identifying antigens using specific antibodies. Western blotting employs gel electrophoresis and solid phase immunoassay methods to detect small amounts of specific proteins in tissue or cellular extracts, with high resolution, specificity and sensitivity. Typically 1 to 5 ng of a medium size protein can be detected. The method is simple, samples can be stored for a long periods in denaturing or non-denaturing buffers, and the results can be easily quantified and compared. For these reasons, Western blotting has become a widely used research tool in field of molecular biology.

在此法中，首先将含有靶蛋白(抗原)的样品用 SDS -聚丙烯酰胺凝胶电泳(SDS-PAGE)

或非变性电泳(native-PAGE)等分离后,通过转印至硝酸纤维素膜或其他膜的表面,然后再通过抗原抗体反应对膜表面的靶蛋白进行特异性检测。

In this method, a sample containing a target protein is spatially resolved by vertical SDS-polyacrylamide gel electrophoresis (SDS-PAGE) or non-denaturing electrophoresis (Native-PAGE), and then transferred to a nitrocellulose or polyvinylidene difluoride (PVDF) membrane *in situ* by horizontal transfer electrophoresis. The spatially resolved proteins become immobilized on the membrane surface and the target protein is detected using antibodies that specifically bind epitopes on that protein.

二、实验方法　Experimental method

免疫印迹的实验程序包括以下 5 个主要步骤：①样品的制备；②凝胶电泳分离样品；③电转移；④封闭膜上的非特异性结合部位；⑤靶蛋白的检测。

(一) 样品的制备　Sample preparation

用于免疫印迹的蛋白样品主要有 3 个来源：①蛋白溶液；②细胞裂解液；③免疫沉淀蛋白。现以如何从贴附型细胞中获取蛋白样品为例介绍样品的制备方法。

There are three main sources of protein samples for immunoblotting：① Protein solution；②Cell lysate；③Immunoprecipitated protein. An example is shown below.

1. 所需试剂　Required reagents

不含 DTT 的 Laemmli 样品缓冲液(裂解液)、1 mol DTT (− 20℃ 冻存)、0.01 mol/L PBS(pH 7.2)。

Laemmli sample buffer (without DTT)，1 mol DTT (store at − 20℃)，0.01 mol/L PBS (pH 7.2)

2. 实验步骤　Protocols

(1) 用适量 PBS 洗涤细胞 2 次,弃干净洗液。

Wash the cells twice with PBS，discard the PBS.

(2) 根据培养细胞的数量加入相应体积的裂解液。通常,每 1 g 细胞(约 10^9 个)加入 1 ml 裂解液,并用细胞刮将细胞刮入离心管中。

Add Laemmli sample buffer to the cells (1 ml per 10^9 cells). Transfer cells to a centrifuge tube with cell scraper.

(3) 加入 10 倍体积的样品缓冲液,强力混匀。

Add 10 times volume of sample buffer and mix vigorously.

(4) 最大强度超声 4 次,每次 15～30 s。在每次超声间隔期,将样品置于冰浴中 15 s。

Lysate cell by ultrasound (ultrasound time 15 to 30 seconds，15 seconds interval on ice).

(5) 70℃孵育至少 5 min。

Incubate at 70℃ for at least 5 minutes.

(6) 10 000×g 离心 10 min,取上清液并转移至新离心管中(若不需立即使用,可将样品在 −20℃ 稳定保存数月)。

Centrifuge at $10\,000 \times g$ for 10 minutes, transfer the supernatant to a new centrifuge tube (the sample can be stored stably at $-20\,℃$ for several months).

3. 附录　Appendix

不含 DTT 的 Laemmli 样品缓冲液（裂解液）：20％ SDS，10％甘油，60 mmol/L Tris（pH 6.8），0.01％溴酚蓝。

Laemmli sample buffer (without DTT)：20％ SDS，10％ glycerol，60 mmol/L Tris (pH 6.8)，0.01％ bromophenol blue.

（二）凝胶电泳　Gel electrophoresis

SDS-PAGE 是分离蛋白最常用的方法，但其他方法如等电聚焦（IEF）、双向电泳（IEF 和 SDS-PAGE)同样可用。在选择电泳方法及电泳条件时应注意以下几个问题：①凝胶电泳缓冲液一定要与印迹膜的类型相匹配；②上样蛋白总量应不能使电泳条带发生变形；③分离胶的浓度要与待分离样品的分子量相适应。SDS-PAGE 的方法请参考常规分子生物学实验方法。

SDS-PAGE is the most common method for separating proteins, but other methods such as isoelectric focusing (IEF) and two-dimensional electrophoresis (IEF and SDS-PAGE) are also available. The following problems should be noted when select electrophoresis methods and electrophoresis conditions：①Gel electrophoresis buffer must match the type of blotting membrane；②The total amount of protein loaded should not deform the electrophoresis band；③The concentration is adapted to the molecular weight of the sample to be separated. For the method of SDS-PAGE electrophoresis, please refer to the conventional molecular biology experimental method.

（三）电转移　Electrotransfer

1. 所需试剂　Required reagents

转移缓冲液、考马斯亮蓝染色液、超纯水。

Transfer buffers，Coomassie brilliant blue staining solution，ultrapure water.

2. 实验步骤（半干电转法）　Protocols (semi-dry electrotransfer)

（1）用超纯水淋洗半干装置的平板电极。

Rinse the electrode plates of the semi-dry appartus with ultrapure water.

（2）将凝胶切成适当大小用于电转，除去无关部分凝胶和未使用的泳道，做好凝胶标记。

Cut gel to appropriate size and mark the gel.

（3）剪取 6 张吸水纸和一张硝酸纤维素（nitrocellulose filter，NC)膜（戴手套操作）。

Cut six sheets of absorbent paper and a nitrocellulose filter (with gloves).

（4）将硝酸纤维素膜浸入超纯水中 2～5 min。

Immerse the nitrocellulose filter into ultrapure water for 2 to 5 minutes.

（5）将吸水纸放入转印缓冲液中浸湿。

Place the absorbent paper in the transfer buffer.

（6）将凝胶、硝酸纤维素膜、滤纸和吸水纸放在平板装置底部，在检查极性、有无气泡后接通电源进行转印。

Place the gel, nitrocellulose filter, filter paper and absorbent paper on the bottom of the flat device, and turn on the power to transfer after checking the polarity and bubbles.

（7）转印结束后，给膜作上标记，用考马斯亮蓝染色液对凝胶进行染色以验证转印的效果。

Mark the nitrocellulose filter and stain with Coomassie brilliant blue solution to verify the effect of the transfer.

3. 附录　Appendix

转移缓冲液：39 mmol/L 甘氨酸，48 mmol/L Tris - HCl，0.037％SDS，20％甲醇。

Transfer buffers：39 mmol/L glycine，48 mmol/L Tris - HCl，0.037％ SDS，20％ methanol.

（四）封闭　Blocking

1. 所需试剂　Required reagents

封闭液。

Blocking solution.

2. 实验步骤　Protocols

（1）将硝酸纤维素膜放在一张干净的滤纸上，室温干燥 30～60 min。

Place the nitrocellulose filter on a clean filter paper and dry at room temperature for 30 to 60 minutes.

（2）将硝酸纤维素膜转移至一平皿中，加入可以浸末滤膜量的封闭液置室温振荡 1～3 h。

Transfer the nitrocellulose filter into the blocking solution, shake at room temperature for 1 to 3 hours.

3. 附录　Appendix

封闭液：5％脱脂奶粉，0.01％的防沫剂（antifoam），0.02％叠氮钠溶于 PBS 中。

Blocking solution：5％ nonfat dry milk，0.01％ antifoam，0.02％ sodium azide in PBS.

（五）抗原抗体反应检测靶蛋白　Antigen and antibody reaction detection target protein

免疫印迹对靶蛋白的检测既可以采用直接法，也可以采用间接法。用标记的一抗直接检测的优点在于：膜的背景较低、简单、快捷，并且减少了交叉反应的机会，但其灵敏度明显低于间接法。除非在特殊情况下使用直接法，通常免疫印迹采用间接法：一抗未标记，而是借助二抗的酶标记进行放大显色，借以显示靶蛋白。

The detection of a target protein in immunoblotting assays can be accomplished using either a direct method or an indirect method. Direct detection using labeled primary antibodies has the advantage of being simple and fast, producing limited cross-reactions with other proteins and low membrane background. The sensitivity of direct methods, however, is significantly lower than indirect methods. For this reason, immunoblotting is usually performed using an indirect detection method：the primary antibody is not labeled, and its location on the blotting membrane is revealed by a colored reaction product generated by an enzyme reporter attached to a secondary antibody.

1. 所需试剂　Required reagents

多克隆抗体、杂交瘤细胞培养上清液、荷瘤小鼠腹水、漂洗液Ⅰ、漂洗液Ⅱ、封闭液、DAB显色液。

Polyclonal antibodies，hybridoma culture supernatant，tumor-bearing mice ascites，Rinse Ⅰ，Rinse Ⅱ，blocking solution，DAB solution.

2. 实验步骤　Protocols

(1) 从封闭液中将膜取出，用 PBS 冲洗 2 次，每次 5 min。

Remove membrane from the blocking solution and rinse twice with PBS for 5 minutes each time.

(2) 加入抗体，抗体用量为 10 ml/15 cm×15 cm 膜，0.5 ml/15 cm×0.5 cm 膜，置一塑料袋中封存。抗体在使用前已经封闭液稀释。

Dilute antibodies with blocking solution. Add diluted antibodies on membrane (10 ml per 15 cm×15 cm，0.5 ml per 15 cm×0.5 cm)，seal in a plastic bag.

(3) 室温下轻轻振荡孵育 1 h。

Incubate the membrane for 1 hour at room temperature with gentle shaking.

(4) 漂洗液Ⅰ洗涤 1 次，10 min。

Rinse the membrane with rinse Ⅰ for 10 minutes.

(5) 将膜转移到另一塑料袋中，加入标记好的且经封闭液稀释的二抗，抗体用量同第二步。

Transfer the membrane to another plastic bag, add the labeled secondary antibodies diluted with blocking solution (10 ml per 15 cm×15 cm，0.5 ml per 15 cm×0.5 cm).

(6) 室温下轻轻振荡孵育 1~2 h。

Incubate for 1 to 2 hours with gentle shaking at room temperature.

(7) 取出滤膜，用大量漂洗液Ⅱ洗涤 3~5 次，每次 10 min，以除去未结合之二抗。

Remove the filter and wash with a large amount of rinse Ⅱ 3 to 5 times for 10 minutes each time to remove unbound secondary antibodies.

(8) 显色：以辣根过氧化物酶标记的抗体为例，常采用二氨基联苯胺(DAB)为底物。将膜置入一适当容器中，按照 10 ml/15 cm×15 cm 膜加入底物溶液，在室温下摇动显色至样品带出现，随后用含 20 mmol/L EDTA 的 PBS 停止反应，室温晾干，保存滤膜，用于结果分析。

Taking horseradish peroxidase-labeled antibodies as an example. DAB is often used as a substrate. Place the membrane in a suitable container, add the substrate solution on membrane (10 ml per 15 cm×15 cm)，shake at room temperature until the bands appear，stop with PBS containing 20 mmol/L EDTA，dry the filter at room temperature for analysis.

3. 附录　Appendix

(1) 一抗的稀释：(用封闭液)

多克隆抗体：1∶100~1∶5 000。

polyclonal antibodies：1：100 to 1：5 000.

杂交瘤细胞培养上清液：不稀释或 1：100 稀释。

Hybridoma culture supernatant：no dilution or 1：100.

荷瘤小鼠腹水：1：1 000～1：10 000。

tumor-bearing mice ascites：1：1 000 to 1：10 000.

(2) 漂洗液Ⅰ:0.01 mol/L PBS (pH7.2)。

Rinse Ⅰ：0.01 mol/L PBS (pH 7.2).

(3) 漂洗液Ⅱ:150 mmol/L NaCl，50 mmol/L Tris‐HCl (pH7.5)。

Rinse Ⅱ：150 mmol/L NaCl，50 mmol/L Tris‐HCl (pH 7.5).

(4) DAB 显色液：称取 6 mg DAB 溶于 10 ml 50 mmol/L 的 Tris‐HCl 中，经滤纸过滤后，加入 10 μl 30%过氧化氢。

DAB solution：weigh 6 mg of DAB，dissolve in 10 ml of 50 mmol/L Tris‐HCl，and filter through filter paper. Add 10 μl of 30% hydrogen peroxide.

第五节 ◎ 组织芯片
Tissue chips

一、概述　Overview

组织芯片(tissue chips)也称组织微阵列(tissue microarrays，TMA)，是生物芯片技术的一个重要分支，是将不同个体组织标本以规则阵列方式排布于同一载体(多为载玻片)上，进行同一指标的原位组织学研究。其最大优势在于芯片上的组织样本实验条件完全一致，有极好的质量控制。是继基因芯片、蛋白质芯片之后出现的又一种重要的生物芯片，主要用于研究同一种基因或蛋白质分子在不同细胞或组织中表达的情况。

Tissue chips，also known as tissue microarrays (TMA)，are an important branch of biochip technology. TMAs comprise arrays of individual tissue samples on single supports (usually glass slides). An advantage of using tissue chips in histological studies is that the experimental conditions of the tissue samples are uniform，thus providing excellent quality control. Tissue chips have become important research tools，following the successes of gene chips and protein chips. For example，they are often used to study the expression of the same gene or protein in different types of cells or tissues.

组织芯片主要用于各种原位组织技术实验中，包括常规形态学观察、各种特殊染色如免疫组织化学、原位杂交(in situ hybridization，ISH)、荧光原位杂交(Fluorescence in situ hybridization，FISH)、原位 PCR、原位 RT‐PCR 和寡核苷酸引物原位 DNA 合成技术(oligonucleotide primed in situ DNA synthesis，PRINS)等。可用于临床和基础研究，如分子诊断、预后指标筛选、治疗靶点定位、抗体和药物筛选、基因和蛋白表达分析等。

TMAs have a wide range of applications in clinical and basic research，including morphological observations，molecular diagnostics，and screening of prognostic indicators， therapeutic target localization, antibody and drug screening, gene and protein expression analysis. They are often used in combination with various detection technologies including, immunohistochemistry (IHC), nucleic acid *in situ* hybridization (ISH), fluorescence *in situ* hybridization (FISH), *in situ* PCR, *in situ* RT - PCR, and oligonucleotide primed *in situ* DNA synthesis (PRINS).

组织芯片的种类包括人的常规石蜡包埋样本的组织芯片、各种实验动物的组织芯片、细胞株及一些病原微生物的芯片等。在已有的石蜡包埋组织芯片的基础上，创建了冷冻组织微阵列技术。随后又将组织学专业知识与数字化病理技术及自动化组织芯片技术相结合，可精准定位所需的组织区域或细胞类型，避免无效组织出现，有助于肿瘤微环境中的病理学研究。

The types of tissue chips include: arrays of conventional paraffin-embedded samples of tissues from humans, various experimental animals, cell strains, and pathogenic microorganisms. Based on the success of paraffin-embedded tissue arrays, chips comprising arrays of frozen tissue have also been developed.

组织芯片与基因芯片配合使用在寻找疾病基因中有很好的互补作用。特别是在肿瘤研究中发挥着重要作用。将基因芯片筛选出的基因作成探针，再将探针与组织芯片中众多的肿瘤组织进行荧光原位杂交，寻找肿瘤发生、发展的相关因素。组织芯片与基因芯片、蛋白质芯片、细胞芯片一起构成了生物芯片系列，使人类第一次能够有效利用成百上千份组织标本，在基因组、转录组和蛋白质组 3 个水平上进行研究。

TMAs are useful complements to genotyping, RNA expression and protein expression microarrays and whole genome/whole exome DNA sequencing in the search for disease genes. For example, each of these technologies already plays important roles in cancer research. Genes screened using genotyping chips or DNA sequencing can be used to develop probes for chip-based quantification of RNA and protein expression, and tumor tissues arrayed on tissue chips can be used to study cell-specific expression of genes (using FISH for detection) related to tumor development. Tissue chips together with gene chips, RNA expression chips, protein chips and tissue chips comprise a series of biochips that enable researchers and clinician to efficiently use hundreds of tissue samples to identify and characterize candidate cancer genes at genomic, transcriptome, proteome and cellular levels.

二、组织芯片构建的原理　TMA construction principle

（1）选取待研究的组织。现在人们利用组织芯片技术对人体各组织均有研究，包括肝脏、前列腺、心脏、乳房和脑组织。医学上常选取一些病变组织进行研究。

Selection of the tissue to be studied. Researchers currently use tissue chip technology to study various tissues of the human body, including liver, prostate, heart, breast and brain tissue. Pathological tissues are often selected for medical research.

（2）经检测后标记出待研究的区域。组织微阵列的检测仪主要是高性能显微镜、荧光显微镜或共聚焦荧光显微镜。适用的检测技术有苏木精-伊红(HE)染色、免疫组织化学染色、原位杂交、荧光原位杂交、原位 PCR、寡核苷酸启动的原位 DNA 合成等。

Identification of tissue regions of interest (ROI) to be studied. Screening of tissue sections mounted on glass slides is usually carried out using high-performance light microscopes, fluorescence microscopes or confocal fluorescence microscopes. Techniques for tissue analysis include: hematoxylin-eosin staining, immunohistochemistry staining, *in situ* hybridization, fluorescence *in situ* hybridization, *in situ* PCR, and oligonucleotide primer *in situ* DNA synthesis. Based on screening tissues using the techniques, tissue ROIs are marked for eventual transfer to tissue chips.

(3) 使用组织芯片点样仪将标记好的组织按设计排列在空白蜡块上。先要利用打孔机在已经标记好的靶位点上进行打孔,将组织芯转入蜡块孔中,重复操作可转入上千个样品组织芯。

Transfer of marked tissue ROIs to wax blocks for sectioning. Marked tissues regions are transferred to an array wax block using a tissue chip spotter. First, a tissue punching machine is used to excise a tissue core within a ROI and this core is then transferred into a hole within an array wax block, an operation be efficiently carried out robotically for thousands of sample tissue cores.

(4) 使用切片机对阵列蜡块进行连续切片即获得组织芯片。根据制作方法来分,微阵列主要有石蜡包埋的组织微阵列和冷冻微阵列两种。后者可以克服前者的多种缺陷,如含醛基的化合物可能损伤 RNA 或使目标抗原结构断裂或破坏抗原抗体结合位点以及石蜡包埋组织中 RNA 的降解。

TMAs are produced by serial sectioning of the array wax blocks using a microtome and transferring these sections to a glass slide. This method can be used to prepare TMAs containing either fixed, paraffin-embedded or frozen tissue cores. Frozen tissues have the advantage of avoiding damage to mRNA or antigenic sites on proteins associated with formaldehyde or glutaraldehyde-based fixation and mRNA degradation often associated with ethanol-fixed tissues.

（杨　娟）

第五章　细胞生存与功能
Survival and function of cells

细胞的增殖、迁移、侵袭和死亡是细胞基本的生命活动,相互关联,相互影响。这些看似独立的细胞基本活动又统一于细胞周期的运行轨道,受着基因的调节,环境信号因子的影响。对细胞生存与功能的检测和机制探讨,与肿瘤发生、发展的研究和抗肿瘤药物的开发应用关系密切。

Proliferation, migration, tissue invasion and death are characteristic cellular activities. Understand the molecular mechanisms underlying cell survival and function is central to the study of cancer and anti-cancer drugs.

第一节 ◎ 细胞增殖与活力
Cell proliferation and cell viability

细胞增殖检测用于分析细胞分裂中细胞数量的变化,进而反应细胞的生长状态及活性,目前广泛应用于肿瘤生物学、分子生物学和药代动力学等领域。细胞增殖检测实验可根据实验方案和目的不同而应用多种不同的实验策略:MTT、XTT、MTS、CCK8 及 SRB 法主要应用于细胞活力、药物作用的毒性等;染料排斥法主要基于活细胞有排斥某些染料如伊红、台盼蓝、苯胺黑等的能力,而死细胞可被着色,适合少量细胞的统计,广泛用于绘制细胞生长曲线等。

Cellular proliferation is an important parameter for many cell and tissue culture experiments. It is often used to characterize the effects of growth factors, assess the biocompatibility of a new materials or test the toxicity of new drugs. Different cell proliferation assays are often used based the experimental designs and objectives of the studies. MTT, XTT, MTS, CCK8 and SRB assays are often used to assess cell viability and toxicity of drug. Dye exclusion tests based on the ability of living cells to exclude certain dyes, such as eosin, trypan blue and aniline black, and is widely used to produce cell growth curves.

一、台盼蓝染色测定细胞活力　Trypan blue exclusion test of cell viability

死细胞和受损细胞的细胞膜通常因缺损而不完整,这样某些染料分子便可穿过细胞膜进入到细胞内部并使细胞被染上相应的颜色。与死细胞和受损细胞不同,活细胞的细胞膜结构完整,能阻止染料进入细胞而拒染(dye exclusion)。台盼蓝(0.4%)便是这样的染料,经台盼蓝染色的死细胞或受损细胞常为浅蓝色。除台盼蓝外,伊红、苯胺黑也是常用的鉴定细胞活力的染料,所不同的是,经伊红和苯胺黑染色的死细胞或受损细胞分别为红色和黑色。

Dye exclusion tests are based on the observation that viable cells do not take up dyes such as trypan blue, but dead cells do. Trypan blue solution (0.4%,) is routinely used as a cell stain to assess cell viability. This test is often performed when counting cells using a hemocytometer during routine subculture and can be performed any time cell viability needs to be determined quickly and accurately.

(一)仪器与试剂　Required equipment and reagents

0.4%台盼蓝溶液,HBSS,血细胞计数板,微量加样器吸头,显微镜,微量加样器,离心管。

0.4% trypan blue solution, HBSS, hemacytometer, pipette tips, light microscopes, pipettes, centrifuge tube.

(二)操作步骤　Protocols

(1) 将贴壁细胞用胰蛋白酶消化后再经 HBSS 洗涤后制备单细胞悬液,并适当调整细胞密度在 10^6 个/ml 左右。

Trypsinize adhesive cells, wash with HBSS to prepare cell suspension, adjust cell density to about 10^6 cells/ml.

(2) 取细胞悬液 0.5 ml 加入离心管中,加入 0.5 ml 0.4%台盼蓝染液,染色 2~3 min。

Transfer 0.5 ml of the cell suspension to a centrifuge tube. Add 0.5 ml of 0.4% trypan blue dye, gently mix and let stand for 2 to 3 minutes.

(3) 用微量加样器吸取少量细胞悬液加入到血细胞计数板上的小室中。

Set up a hemocytometer and cover slip. Place one drop of the cell suspension onto the hemocytometer.

(4) 显微镜下分别数出死细胞和总细胞数,计算细胞活力。

Observe the cells under a light microscope at low magnification. Count the total number of cells and the number of stained cells.

(5) 结果判定:死细胞能被台盼蓝染色,镜下可见其为浅蓝色的细胞,活细胞不能被染色,镜下呈无色透明状。

细胞活力(%)=(总细胞数-着色的死细胞数)÷总细胞数×100%

Viewed under the microscope, only dead cells appear blue in color.

Cell viability (%)=(total number of cells-number of stained cells)/total number of cells×100%

(三)注意事项　Notes

(1) 和台盼蓝溶液混合后的细胞悬液不可放置时间过长,因为活细胞对染料也有一定摄取能力,若时间太长,活细胞也会被染色。

Cell suspensions containing trypan blue should not be let to sit for long periods of time，because living cells will slowly absorb dyes used in dye exclusion assays. If the time of exposure to a dye is too long，living cells will also be stained.

（2）细胞悬液和台盼蓝溶液的用量可根据实验条件及要求进行必要调整。

The ratio of cell suspension to trypan blue solution can be adjusted according to the experimental conditions and requirements.

（3）血细胞计数板用完后要及时用水、70%乙醇认真清洗计数板和盖玻片，并用擦镜纸擦干后保存。

After use，the hemocytometer and cover slip should be rinsed，first with water，and then with 70% ethanol，and dried by wiping with lens paper.

二、MTT 或 CCK8 法测细胞相对数目和相对活力　MTT and CCK - 8 cell viability assay

四唑盐比色实验是一种常用的检测细胞存活与生长状况的方法，实验所用的显色剂是一种能接受氢原子的染料，化学名为 3 -（4,5 -二甲基噻唑- 2)- 2,5 -二苯基四氮唑溴盐(3-(4,5-dimethylthiazol-2-yl)-2,5-diphenyltetrazolium bromide，MTT)，商品名是噻唑蓝。活细胞，特别是增殖期的细胞可通过线粒体代谢过程中产生的琥珀酸脱氢酶的作用，使外源性淡黄色的 MTT 被还原为蓝紫色的结晶物甲臜(formazan)并沉积在细胞中，其形成量与活细胞数呈正相关。利用 DMSO 或酸化异丙醇进一步溶解细胞中的紫色结晶物，在酶标仪或分光光度计波长 570 nm 处测定吸光度(optical density，OD)，可间接反映出活细胞数量的变化情况。

Yellow MTT ［3-(4，5-dimethylthiazol-2-yl)-2，5-diphenyltetrazolium bromide］，a tetrazole，is converted to a purple formazan in mitochondria of living cells. Mitochondrial dehydrogenases of viable cells cleave the MTT tetrazolium ring，yielding purple formazan，which is insoluble in aqueous solutions. This reductive cleavage takes place only in living cells. The absorbance of formazan at 570 nm is measured using a spectrophotometer after solubilization in DMSO.

2 -（2 -甲氧基- 4 -硝苯基)- 3 -(4 -硝苯基)- 5 -(2,4 -二磺基苯)- 2H -四唑单钠盐)［2-(2-methoxy-4-nitrophenyl)-3-(4-nitrophenyl)-5-(2， 4-disulfophenyl)-2H-tetrazolium，WST-8]是一种类似于 MTT 的化合物，在电子耦合剂存在的情况下，可以被线粒体内的一些脱氢酶还原生成橙黄色的甲臜，具有高度水溶性(图 5 - 1)。生成橙黄色甲臜的数量和活细胞的数量成正比。Cell Counting Kit - 8(CCK - 8)检测法是一种基于 WST - 8 广泛应用于细胞增殖和细胞毒性的快速高灵敏度检测法，可用于药物筛选、细胞增殖测定、细胞毒性测定、肿瘤药敏等试验。

Cell Counting Kit-8 (CCK-8) allows convenient assays using WST-8 ［2-(2-methoxy-4-nitrophenyl)-3-(4-nitrophenyl)-5-(2，4-disulfophenyl)-2H-tetrazolium］，which produces a water-soluble formazan dye in the presence of an electron carrier. WST-8 is reduced by dehydrogenases in the cells giving an orange colored formazan，which is soluble in the tissue culture medium(Fig. 5 - 1). The amount of the formazan dye generated by dehydrogenases in cells is directly proportional to the number of living cells.

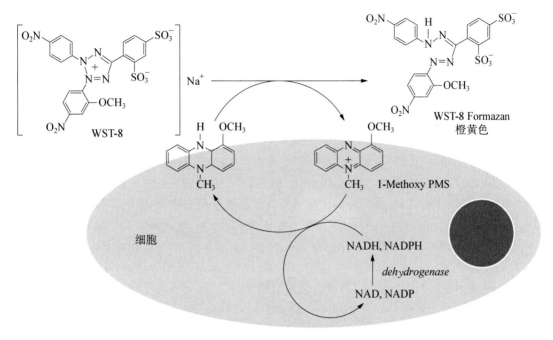

图 5-1　WST-8检测细胞活力的原理

Fig. 5-1　Principle of the cell viability detection with WST-8

（一）仪器与试剂　Required equipment and reagents

96 孔细胞培养板、RPMI 1640 培养基(10%FBS)、5 mg/ml MTT 溶液、DMSO、CCK-8 溶液、酶标仪。

96-well cell culture plates, RPMI 1640 medium (10% FBS), 5 mg/ml MTT solution, DMSO, CCK-8 solution, microplate spectrophotometer.

（二）操作步骤　Protocols

1. MTT 检测法　MTT assay

(1) 取对数生长期的贴附型细胞经消化、洗涤后以一定密度接种在平底 96 孔细胞培养板上，每组设 3 个平行孔，每孔 200 μl。

Seed cells into a 96-well cell culture plate (three parallel wells in each group, 200 μl per well) at a certain density.

(2) 将 96 孔细胞培养板移入细胞培养箱，37℃、5%CO₂ 和饱和湿度条件下培养。

Put 96-well cell culture plate in a humidified incubator for 24 h (37℃, 5% CO₂).

(3) 向培养板加入 10 μl 不同浓度的待测物质。

Add 10 μl of various concentrations of substances to be tested to the plate.

(4) 将培养板在培养箱孵育一段适当的时间(例如，6、12、24 或 48 h)。

Incubate the plate for an appropriate length of time (such as 6, 12, 24 and 48 hours) in the incubator.

(5) 每孔加入 20 μl MTT 溶液(5 mg/ml)，继续孵育 4 h 后终止培养。将培养板

1 000 r/min 离心 5 min 后,从每孔小心吸弃上清液 100 μl,再加入 DMSO 150 μl,振荡 15 min,以使结晶物充分溶解。

Add 20 μl of 5 mg/ml MTT solution to each well. Include one set of wells with MTT but no cells, as a control. Return the plate to incubator for no more than 4 hours. Centrifuge the plate to pellet the cells (1 000 r/min, 5 min), discard supernatant, add 150 μl DMSO, agitate the cells on orbital shaker for 15 min to solubilize the MTT formazan.

(6) 选择 570 nm 波长,在酶标仪上测定各孔的 OD 值,记录结果。

Measure the OD value at 570 nm using a microplate spectrophotometer.

2. CCK - 8 法　CCK - 8 assay

(1) 取对数生长期的贴附型细胞经消化、洗涤后以一定密度接种在平底 96 孔细胞培养板上,每组设 3 个平行孔,每孔 200 μl。将培养板放在培养箱中培养 24 h(37℃,5% CO_2)。

Seed cells into a 96-well plate (three parallel wells in each group, 200 μl per well) at a specific density. Incubate the plate for 24 hours in a humidified incubator (37℃, 5% CO_2).

(2) 向培养板加入 10 μl 不同浓度的待测物质。

Add 10 μl of various concentrations of substances to be tested to the plate.

(3) 将培养板在培养箱孵育一段适当的时间(例如,6、12、24 或 48 h)。

Continue to incubate the plate for an appropriate length of time (such as 6, 12, 24 and 48 hours) in the humidified incubator.

(4) 向每孔加入 10 μl CCK - 8 溶液。

Add 10 μl of CCK - 8 solution to each well of the plate.

(5) 将培养板在培养箱内孵育 1~4 h。

Incubate the plate for 1 to 4 hours in the incubator.

(6) 用酶标仪测定在 450 nm 处的 OD 值。

Measure the OD value at 450 nm using a microplate spectrophotometer.

(三) 注意事项　Notes

(1) 依据实验目的、细胞种类、细胞的生长习性选择适当的细胞接种密度和培养时间长短。一般情况下,96 孔细胞培养板每孔最多可以生长 1×10^5 个细胞,切不可接种密度太高,致使培养终止前细胞过满,影响实验的区分度。

The incubation time varies with the type and number of cells in the wells. Generally, the seeding density should not be too high, which will cause the cells to be too full before the culture is terminated, affecting the results of the experiment.

(2) 加入试剂时,建议斜贴着培养板壁加,避免产生气泡,气泡会干扰吸光度的读数。

Since bubbles can interfere with the spectrophotometric measurements, avoid producing bubbles in the wells when pipetting.

(3) 设空白对照孔。空白对照孔不加细胞只加培养基,其他步骤与实验孔相同,比色时以此孔调零。

Set a blank control well containing no cells and processed in the same way as the wells containing cells.

三、细胞的分裂指数　Mitotic index

分裂指数是衡量体外培养细胞生长增殖状况的重要指标,常用细胞群体中分裂细胞所占的百分比来表示。分裂指数是测定细胞周期的一个重要指标,与生长曲线有一定的联系,如随着分裂指数的不断提高,细胞也就进入了对数生长期。同时,分裂指数也是不同实验研究选择细胞的重要依据。

Mitotic index assays provide an alternative method to measure cellular proliferation. In addition to providing a simple measurement of the percentage of cells undergoing mitosis, the mitotic index provides important information for cell cycle research and markers for the selection of subsets of cells.

（一）仪器与试剂　Required equipment and reagents

细胞培养皿、盖玻片、细胞培养基(如含 10% FBS 的 RPMI 1640)、0.25%胰蛋白酶液(含 0.02% EDTA)、甲醇、冰醋酸、吉姆萨(Giemsa)染液、PBS 溶液,光学显微镜。

Cell culture dishes, coverslip, RPMI 1640 medium (10%FBS), 0.25% trypsin solution (0.02% EDTA), methanol, glacial acetic acid, Giemsa staining solution, PBS, light microscope.

（二）操作步骤　Protocols

(1) 将消化、洗涤后的贴附型细胞以一定密度接种至内含盖玻片的培养皿中。

Seed cells into a cell culture dish (containing cover slips) at a certain density.

(2) 置细胞培养箱中培养 48 h,使细胞贴附在盖玻片上生长。

Incubate the plate for 48 hours in the cell culture incubator.

(3) 取出盖玻片,PBS 漂洗 3 min,固定液(甲醇∶冰醋酸＝3∶1 体积比)固定 30 min,Giemsa 染液染色 10 min 后用水冲洗。

Remove the coverslips, wash with PBS for 3 minutes, fix cells with methanol and acetic acid (3∶1 volume ratio), stain with Giemsa staining solution for 10 minutes, and wash with water.

(4) 镜检,计数分裂期的细胞数目和总细胞数目。

Observe the coverslips under a light microscope. Count the number of cells undergoing mitosis and the total cells.

(5) 计算结果如下。

分裂指数＝分裂细胞数／总细胞数×100%

Mitotic index＝number of cells in mitosis/total cells×100%

（三）注意事项　Notes

(1) 操作时动作要轻,以免使盖玻片上的细胞脱落。

Handle coverslips gently to prevent cells from falling off.

(2) 细胞接种密度、培养时间由细胞的种类及生长习性决定。

Optimal cell density and culture time are cell type-dependent.

四、集落形成实验　Colony formation assay

集落(克隆)形成实验是检验细胞存活率和增殖能力的有效指标。集落或克隆是指单个细胞在体外经 6 代以上增殖后所形成的细胞群体,直径常在 0.3~1.0 mm。正常细胞在体外培养时由于常需附着在坚硬的玻璃或塑料表面才能生长,而转化的或恶变的肿瘤细胞却常常丧失附着依赖生长的特性,可在软琼脂或甲基纤维素中以集落的方式生长。通过对集落的计数,不仅可以了解细胞的生存增殖能力,而且还可用于评价肿瘤细胞对抗肿瘤药物的敏感性、肿瘤放射生物学研究。常用的集落形成实验主要有平板集落形成实验和软琼脂集落形成实验,此处主要介绍软琼脂集落形成实验。

Colony formation assays are a convenient method for quantifying cell survival and proliferation for progeny of single cells. Single-cell cloning often involves the isolation and culture of cells in single colonies formed by the proliferation of single cells for more than 6 generations in *in vitro* culture. Colony diameters are typically 0.3 to 1.0 mm. When cultured *in vitro*, normal cells often need to attach to hard glass or plastic surfaces to grow. By contrast, transformed or malignant tumor cells have often lost their attachment-dependent properties, allowing growth and colony in soft agar or methyl cellulose.

(一) 仪器与试剂　Required equipment and reagents

24 孔细胞培养板、细胞培养基(如含 10% FBS 的 RPMI 1640)、0.25% 胰蛋白酶液(含 0.02% EDTA)、琼脂粉、倒置显微镜

24-well cell culture plate, RPMI 1640 medium (10% FBS), 0.25% trypsin/0.02% EDTA solution, agarose, inverted microscope.

(二) 操作步骤　Protocols

(1) 制备细胞悬液:取对数生长期贴附型细胞经消化、洗涤后用培养基根据实验要求稀释调整细胞密度,待用。

Prepare cell suspension: Harvest cells by trypsinization and adjust the cell density according to the experimental requirements.

(2) 制备底层琼脂:用超纯水配制 5% 的琼脂,高压灭菌后待温度降至 50℃,加入预温的 9 倍体积培养基稀释,混匀后迅速加入 24 孔细胞培养板(每孔 0.8 ml),室温待琼脂凝固。

Prepare the bottom of agar: Prepare 5% agar with ultrapure water, reduce the temperature to 50℃ after high-pressure sterilization, add pre-warmed 9-fold volume medium, gently mix. Add 0.8 ml mixture into each well (24-well cell culture plate), and allow agar mixture to solidify at room temperature.

(3) 制备上层琼脂:取 0.6 ml 保温于 50℃的 5% 的琼脂与 9.6 ml 细胞悬液迅速混匀后立即加入到铺有底层琼脂的 24 孔培养板中,每孔 0.8 ml,室温待上层琼脂凝固。

Prepare the upper layer of Agar: Mix 0.6 ml of 5% agar solution (heat preservation at 50℃) and 9.6 ml cell suspension, add mixture to 24-well cell culture plate with bottom agar, 0.8 ml per well, allow agar mixture to solidify at room temperature.

(4) 将 24 孔培养板在细胞培养箱中培养 7~14 d。

Incubate the cells for 7 to 14 days in the incubator (37℃ and 5% CO_2).

（5）倒置显微镜下计数集落数目，按下面公式计算结果。

集落数＝n 个孔的细胞集落数总和÷孔数（n）

集落形成率＝（集落数÷接种细胞总数）×100%

Count the number of colonies under inverted microscope and calculate the results according to the following formula.

Number of colonies＝the total number of cell colonies/the number of wells（n）

Colony formation rate＝（colony number/total number of seeded cells）×100%.

（三）注意事项　Notes

（1）制备琼脂时尽量避免气泡和局部结块的产生。

Avoid bubbles and local caking during the preparation of agar.

（2）琼脂与完全培养基混合温度不要超过 50℃，与细胞悬液混合时的温度不要超过 40℃，以免降解培养基的营养成分和损伤细胞。

The mixing temperature of agar and complete medium should not exceed 50℃, and the temperature of mixing with cell suspension should not exceed 40℃, so as not to degrade the nutrient composition of the medium and damage the cells.

第二节 ◎ 细胞周期
Cell cycle

一、概述　Overview

细胞周期时间指细胞一个世代所经历的时间，即从一次细胞分裂结束到下一次分裂结束所经历的时间，反映了细胞增殖速度。测定群体细胞周期的方法很多，主要有同位素标记法、细胞计数法和流式细胞仪测定等。这里主要介绍利用 5-溴 2'-脱氧尿嘧啶核苷（5-bromo-2'-deoxyuridine，BrdU）渗入法测定细胞周期。

Cell cycle time refers to the time experienced by one generation of cells, that is, from the end of one cell division to the end of the next division, which reflects the rate of cell proliferation. Using BrdU staining of cells for cell cycle analysis is one method.

BrdU 加入培养基后，可代替胸腺嘧啶核苷掺入到所复制的 DNA 新链中，经过一轮复制，每条染色单体的一条 DNA 链均含有 BrdU，但经染色后染色体却仍为深染。经过两个细胞周期后，细胞中两条单链均含 BrdU 的 DNA 将占总数的 1/2，反映在中期染色体上表现为其中的一条单体浅染。但若经历了 3 个周期，则约一半染色体的两条单体均浅染，另一半为一深一浅。这样，通过统计分裂相中各期的比例，就可算出细胞周期的值。

二、仪器与试剂　Required equipment and reagents

培养瓶、微量加样器、离心管、30W 紫外灯、细胞培养基（如含 10% FBS 的 RPMI 1640）、0.25%胰蛋白酶液（含 0.02% EDTA）、HBSS、BrdU（1.0 mg/ml）溶液、甲醇、冰醋酸、

Giemsa 染液、秋水仙素、2×柠檬酸钠 SSC 液、显微镜、离心机。

Culture flask, pipettes, centrifuge tubes, 30 W ultraviolet lamp, RPMI 1640 medium (10% FBS), 0.25% trypsin/0.02% EDTA solution, HBSS, BrdU (1.0 mg/ml) solution, methanol, glacial acetic acid, Giemsa staining solution, colchicine, 2×SSC solution, light microscope, centrifuge.

三、操作步骤　Protocols

（1）取对数生长期贴附型细胞经消化、洗涤后以一定密度种植在培养瓶或 96 孔细胞培养板中。

Seed cells onto a 96-well plate or a culture flask.

（2）细胞生长至对数生长期时，向培养液中加入 BrdU，使最终浓度为 10 μg/ml，培养 44～54 h。

Add BrdU to the culture solution (the final concentration of 10 μg/ml). Incubate the cells for 44 to 54 hours in incubator (37℃, 5% CO_2).

（3）加入秋水仙素，终浓度为 0.1 μg/ml，继续培养 4～6 h。

Add colchicine to the culture solution (the final concentration of 0.1 μg/ml). Incubate the cells for 4 to 6 hours.

（4）常规消化细胞至离心管中，注意培养上清液的漂浮细胞也收集到离心管中。

Digest the cells and transfer all cells into the centrifuge tube.

（5）按照常规染色体制备方法制片。

Make a slide according the method of chromosome preparation.

（6）将染色体玻片置于 56℃水浴锅盖上，铺上 2% SSC 液，距紫外灯管 6 cm 处紫外照射 30 min。

Put the chromosome slide on the top of water bath (56℃), add 2×SSC solution on the slide, and irradiate with 30 W ultraviolet for 30 min.

（7）弃去 2% SSC 液，立即用 4℃左右的流水冲洗。

Discard the 2% SSC solution and wash immediately with water (4℃).

（8）Giemsa 液染色 5～10 min，流水冲洗，干燥后镜检。

Stain with Giemsa staining solution for 5 to 10 minutes, wash with water, and observe under the microscope.

（9）镜检 100 个分裂象，统计第一、二、三、四细胞期分裂指数。

Examine 100 mitotic phases, count the mitotic indices of the first, second, third and fourth cell phases.

（10）根据下式计算细胞周期。

细胞周期(Tc) = 48/{(M1＋2M2＋3M3＋4M4)/100}(h)

Calculate the cell cycle.

Cell cycle (Tc) = 48/{(M1＋2M2＋3M3＋4M4)/100}(h)

四、注意事项 Notes

（1）秋水仙素加入的时机因细胞的类型、生长条件有所差异。

Addition of colchicine to the cells varies depending on cell type and growth conditions.

（2）加入 BrdU 后应避光培养。

After adding BrdU，cells should be protected from light to avoid photobleaching.

第三节 ◎ 细胞死亡
Cell death

细胞死亡可能是机体新陈代谢的自然过程，也可能是如疾病、局部损伤或细胞参与的有机体死亡。细胞死亡的种类很多，其中凋亡和自噬为程序性细胞死亡，而坏死是由于感染或损伤而发生的病理性过程。

Cell death may be the result of the natural process of new cells replacing old cells，or external factors as disease，localized injury，or the death of the organism of which the cells are part．Two types of programmed cell death，apoptosis and autophagy，have been shown to play important roles the development of organisms．By contrast，necrosis，a non-intrinsic process，occurs in response to infection or injury.

一、细胞凋亡 Apoptosis

可根据死亡细胞在形态学、生物化学和分子生物学上的差别，鉴别凋亡和坏死。细胞凋亡的检测方法有很多，常用的有 TUNEL 法和 Hoechst/PI 染色法等。

Apoptosis and necrosis can be distinguished based on differences in morphology，biochemistry and molecular biology of dying cells．Methods used to detect apoptosis include，TUNEL and Hoechst 33342/propidium iodide（Hoechst/PI）double staining.

（一）TUNEL 法 TUNEL assay

脱氧核糖核苷酸衍生物地高辛［(digoxigenin)-11-dUTP］在 TdT 酶的作用下，可以掺入到凋亡细胞双链或单链 DNA 的 $3'-OH$ 末端，与 dATP 形成异多聚体，并可与连接了报告酶（过氧化物酶或碱性磷酸酶）的抗地高辛抗体结合。在适合底物存在下，过氧化物酶可产生很强的颜色反应，特异精准的定位出正在凋亡的细胞，因而可在普通光学显微镜下进行观察。此即为脱氧核苷酸末端转移酶介导的 dUTP 缺口末端标记（terminal deoxynucleotidyl transferase-dUTP nick end labeling，TUNEL）法。

Apoptosis is the most intensively studied form of programmed cell death and is characterized by specific biochemical and morphological changes，which can be detected by several methods．Nuclear changes correlated with apoptosis include specific patterns of DNA fragmentation that can be detected by terminal deoxynucleotidyl transferase-dUTP nick end labeling（TUNEL）assay，specifically by the transfer of labelled dNTP to $3'-OH$

ends of DNA fragments by terminal deoxynucleotidyltransferase.

1. 仪器与试剂　Required equipment and reagents

0.2% TritonX-100、TUNEL 检测试剂盒(包含 10×TdT 酶浓缩液、荧光素标记的 1× dUTP、转化剂 POD)、DAB 试剂盒、3%过氧化氢甲醇、甲醛、PBS、恒温箱。

0.2% TritonX - 100，TUNEL detection kit，DAB kit，3% H_2O_2 carbinol，formaldehyde，PBS，incubator.

2. 操作步骤　Protocols

(1) 样品处理:在标有实验组,阳性对照组和阴性对照组的切片上滴加 4%不含甲醇的甲醛,室温固定 10 min。弃去甲醛,用 PBS 洗 2 次,每次 5 min。

Fix cells (on slides) with 4% formaldehyde (methanol-free) for 10 minutes at room temperature. Discard formaldehyde and wash twice with PBS for 5 minutes each time.

(2) 封闭:用滤纸擦去切片周围多余的 PBS,滴加 3%过氧化氢,室温孵育 10 min,用 PBS 洗 2 次,每次 5 min。

Incubate slides with 3% H_2O_2 for 10 minutes at room temperature. Discard the H_2O_2 and wash twice with PBS for 5 minutes each time.

(3) 细胞通透化:去尽 PBS 后,滴加 100 μl 由 PBS 配制的 0.2% Triton X - 100,于湿盒中室温孵育 5 min。孵育结束后,弃去 Triton X - 100,PBS 洗 2 次,每次 5 min。

Incubate slides with 100 μl 0.2% Triton X - 100 for 5 minutes in humidified chamber at room temperature. Discard the TritonX - 100 and wash twice with PBS for 5 minutes each time.

(4) TUNEL 反应:按照试剂盒说明书根据实验实际用量配制好标记反应体系。实验组和阳性对照组滴加 50 μl 标记反应混合物,阴性对照组滴加 50 μl 标记溶液,避光孵育 30 min。孵育结束后,用 PBS 洗 2 次,每次 10 min。

Treat the experimental group and the positive control group with 50 μl labeled reaction mixture, and treat the negative control group with 50 μl labeled solution. Incubate for 30 minutes in dark. Wash slides twice with PBS for 10 minutes each time.

(5) POD 转化:擦去周围多余的 PBS,每张切片滴加 50 μl 的转化剂 POD,避光反应 30 min。孵育结束后,PBS 洗 2 次,每次 5 min。

Add 50 μl POD per slide, incubate for 30 minutes in dark and wash twice with PBS for 5 minutes each time.

(6) DAB 染色:取出载玻片,用滤纸擦去周围多余的 PBS。滴加新鲜配制的 DAB 工作液,显微镜下观察背景颜色变化,控制显色时间。底面出现适量黄色时,将载玻片放入盛有蒸馏水的切片缸内,纯水洗终止显色。

Add fresh DAB working solution, use the purified water to stop coloration.

(7) 镜检。

Observe the slides under the microscope.

（二）Hoechst/PI 染色法　Hoechst 33342/propidium iodide（Hoechst/PI）double staining method

细胞发生凋亡时,细胞膜的通透性增加,程度介于正常细胞和坏死细胞之间,利用这一特点,被检细胞悬液用荧光素染色后,通过流式细胞仪检测细胞中的荧光强度来区分正常细胞、坏死细胞和凋亡细胞。

Flow cytometry can be used to detect the fluorescence intensities in cell suspensions to distinguish normal cells, necrotic cells and apoptotic cells.

采用 Hoechst/PI 染色法,正常细胞对染料有抗拒性,荧光染色很浅;凋亡细胞主要摄取 Hoechst 染料,呈现强蓝色荧光;而坏死细胞主要摄取碘化丙啶(PI)而呈强的红色荧光。

Following Hoechst/PI staining, normal cells are only weakly stained, apoptotic cells are preferentially stained by Hoechst 33342 and show strong blue fluorescence, and necrotic cells are preferentially stained by propidium iodide (PI) and show strong red fluorescence.

1. 仪器与试剂 Required equipment and reagents

Hoechst 33342(0.1 mg/ml)、PI(1 mg/ml)、PBS、细胞培养基(如添加有 10%FBS 的 RPMI 1640)、荧光显微镜。

Hoechst 33342(0.1 mg/ml), PI (1 mg/ml), PBS, RPMI 1640 medium (10% PBS), fluorescence microscope.

2. 操作步骤 Protocols

(1) 用 PBS 清洗细胞后,加入含 2%过氧化氢的 PBS,于室温反应 5 min。再用 PBS 洗 2 次,每次 5 min。

Wash the cells with PBS, incubate with 2% H_2O_2 (in PBS) for 5 minutes at room temperature. Wash with PBS twice again, 5 minutes each time.

(2) 1 ml 细胞悬液(细胞密度为 $1×10^6$ 个/ml)中,加入 10 μl Hoechst 33342 储存液,混匀。

Add 10 μl Hoechst 33342 to the 1 ml cell suspension (cell density: $1×10^6$ cells/ml).

(3) 置于 37℃温育 5～15 min。

Incubate the cells for 5 to 15 minutes at 37℃.

(4) 将细胞置于冰上冷却后,于 4℃离心,去除上清液。

Cool the cells on ice, centrifuge at 4℃, and discard supernatant.

(5) 将细胞重新悬浮于 1 ml PBS 中,加入 5 μl PI 储存液,混匀,37℃复染 10～15 min。

Suspend the cells with 1 ml PBS and mix with 5 μl PI. Incubate the cells for 5 to 15 minutes at 37℃.

(6) PBS 洗涤,制片,用荧光显微镜观察分析。

Wash the cells with PBS, drop cell suspension on the slides, observe under fluorescence microscope.

3. 注意事项 Notes

(1) 整个操作动作要尽量轻柔,勿用力吹打细胞。

The whole operation should be gentle as far as possible, do not blow hard on the cells.

(2) 操作时注意避光,反应完毕后尽快在 1 h 内检测。

Pay attention to avoid light during operation, observe the results within one hour after incubation with PI.

二、细胞自噬　Autophagy or autophagocytosis

细胞自噬（autophagy or autophagocytosis）是细胞在自噬相关基因（autophagyrelated gene，Atg）的调控下利用溶酶体降解自身受损的细胞器和大分子物质的过程。自噬主要被分为 3 类：巨自噬（macroautophagy）、微自噬（microautophagy）和分子伴侣介导的（chaperone-mediated autophagy，CMA）。通常所讲的自噬就是指巨自噬，电子显微镜下能观察到双层膜包裹胞质成分的"自噬体"。微自噬是指溶酶体主动、直接吞噬胞质成分。分子伴侣介导的自噬则是指一些分子伴侣，如热休克蛋白 70（HSP 70），能帮助未折叠蛋白转位入溶酶体。

Autophagy, also called autophagocytosis, is a process by which worn, abnormal, or malfunctioning cellular components are degraded in lysosomes. Autophagy serves a housekeeping function by enabling the breakdown and recycling of cellular materials and helps balance energy demands during periods of stress. Three types of autophagy have been described: macroautophagy, microautophagy, and chaperone-mediated autophagy. Cells rely primarily on macroautophagy, in which worn or damaged cellular organelles and molecules are engulfed by autophagosomes (vesicles with double membranes), which deliver their contents to lysosomes, where they are degraded). In microautophagy, cellular components are engulfed directly via invaginations of the lysosomal membrane. Chaperone-mediated autophagy is a selective process, whereby the hsc70 chaperone protein binds proteins containing a specific amino acid motif and delivers these to lysosomes, where they are translocated across the membrane via a receptor-mediated process.

目前，检测细胞自噬最常用的 4 种技术分别为：①利用电子显微镜直接观察自噬小体和自噬溶酶体的形态和数量，需要使用透射电子显微镜。其中，自噬体是由包裹未吞噬降解的胞质物质、细胞器的双层膜结构组成，而自噬溶酶体由单层膜结构组成，其中包裹着处于不同降解阶段的胞质成分；②通过丹磺酰尸胺（Dansylcadaverine，MDC）染色检测细胞自噬。MDC 是一种荧光色素，是嗜酸性染色剂，通常被用于检测自噬体形成的特异性标记染色剂，可将正常细胞均匀染成黄绿色荧光，而自噬细胞染色质浓缩，细胞核碎裂成点状，被染成大小不一、致密浓染的绿色颗粒；③LC3 翻译后加工及脂化修饰，可以通过免疫染色或免疫印迹技术检测 LC3 Ⅰ，LC3 Ⅱ和 p62 的蛋白表达水平；④荧光蛋白标记的 LC3 来检测自噬流。直接通过将 LC3 与荧光蛋白融合，通过荧光蛋白的表达变化来指示 LC3 的蛋白表达。如 GFP－LC3 病毒系统可高效感染目的细胞，表达 GFP－LC3，可在荧光显微镜下实时观察感染后细胞自噬的整体水平。

本章将介绍 LC3 表达的免疫染色检测。

This chapter will introduce immunohistochemical detection of LC3.

（一）仪器与试剂　Required equipment and reagents

PBS、4% 多聚甲醛、LC3 抗体、0.5% Triton X－100、3% BSA、FITC 标记的 IgG、DAPI、PI、激光扫描共聚焦显微镜。

PBS，4% paraformaldehyde，LC3 antibody，0. 5% Triton X - 100，3% BSA，IgG (FITC labeled)，DAPI，PI，Laser scanning confocal microscope.

（二）**操作步骤　Protocols**

（1）将细胞接种在盖玻片上,培养 2～4 h。

Seed cells on cover slides and culture for 2 to 4 hours.

（2）用 PBS 浸洗,然后用 4% 多聚甲醛固定 20 min。

Wash with PBS and fix with 4% paraformaldehyde for 20 minutes.

（3）用 PBS 浸洗 2 次,再用 0. 5% Triton X - 100 处理细胞 5 min。

Wash with PBS twice, and treat with 0. 5% Triton X - 100 for 5 minutes.

（4）PBS 浸洗后用 3% BSA 孵育 30 min。

Wash with PBS and incubate with 3% BSA for 30 minutes.

（5）加入 LC3 抗体(1：100),在 4℃ 条件下过夜。

Add LC3 antibody (1：100) and overnight at 4℃.

（6）用 PBS 清洗 3 次,然后加入 FITC 标记的 IgG(1：100),在 37℃ 条件下孵育 30 min。

Wash with PBS 3 times, add FITC-labeled IgG (1：100) and incubate for 30 minutes at 37℃.

（7）PBS 清洗后,用 DAPI 或 PI(1：1 000)染细胞核。

Wash with PBS, stain with DAPI or PI (1：1 000).

（8）磷酸缓冲甘油封片,在共聚焦激光扫描显微镜下观察 LC3 阳性结构。

Observe LC3 positive structure under laser scanning confocal microscopy.

（三）**注意事项　Notes**

在细胞铺展充分时染色,可降低 LC3 阳性结构的重叠。

Try to spread the cells adequately, which can avoid the overlap of LC3 positive structures.

第四节 ◉ 细胞迁移和细胞侵袭
Cell migration and cell invasion

一、细胞迁移　Cell migration

细胞迁移通常是细胞或细胞簇在化学信号刺激下从一个区域移动到另一个区域的运动,是实现伤口愈合、细胞分化、胚胎发育和肿瘤转移等功能的关键。比如创伤愈合,细胞迁移的时候,以侧向运动为主,细胞划痕实验(wound healing assay)很好地模拟了这种运动形式,是很好的细胞迁移模型。

Cell migration is the movement of cells or cell clusters from one area to another generally in response to a chemical signal, is central to achieving functions such as wound repair, cell differentiation, embryonic development and the metastasis of tumors. The wound healing assay is used to investigate cell migration.

细胞划痕实验是指在单层培养细胞中,通过针或枪尖划痕使小片细胞损伤脱落,进而借助显微镜对细胞再次迁入并填充缺口处进行适时观察。根据细胞类型、培养条件及划痕大小的不同,迁移时间也会有所差异。

(一)仪器与试剂 Required equipment and reagents

6 孔细胞培养板、RPMI 1640 培养基、PBS、培养箱。

6-well cell culture plates, RPMI 1640 medium, PBS, incubator.

(二)操作步骤 Protocols

(1) 先用记号笔在 6 孔细胞培养板背后,用直尺比着,均匀画横线,每隔 0.5～1.0 cm 一道,横穿过孔。每孔至少 5 条线。

Use the marker pen to draw some lines on the back of the 6-well cell culture plate, compare with a ruler, evenly gap 0.5 to 1.0 cm. At least 5 lines per well.

(2) 每孔加入约 2×10^6 个细胞。

Add 2×10^6 cells into each well.

(3) 当细胞生长达到 100%融合(24～48 h)用枪头比着直尺,尽量垂至于背后的横线划痕,枪头要垂直,不能倾斜。

When cells reach 100% confluency (usually 24 to 48 h), create wound with a pipette tip.

(4) 用 PBS 洗细胞 3 次,去除划下的细胞,加入无血清培养基。

Wash the plates three times and replace with the serum-free medium.

(5) 放入 37℃ 5% CO_2 培养箱培养。按 0、6、12、24 h 取样,拍照。

Return cells to a 37℃ cell culture incubator. Acquire both phase contrast and images every 6 hours by matching the wounded region until the wound has completely closed (usually about 24 hours).

二、细胞侵袭 Cell invasion

细胞迁移和侵袭能力的异常与癌症、动脉粥样硬化和关节炎等疾病关系密切。细胞侵袭试验亦被广泛应用于细胞行为研究和肿瘤细胞转移的评估等。细胞侵袭检测最常用的检测方法是 Transwell 侵袭实验(Transwell invasion assay)。

Abnormal cell migration and invasion can contribute to disease progression, including for cancer, atheroscelerosis and arthritis. Research on cell invasion is an important area of medical research and has been facilitated by the development of invasion assays. For example, invasion assays are widely used to investigate the cellular mechanisms of and potential for tumor cell metastasis. Many methods are currently available to study cell invasion. Among these, the Transwell invasion assay is one of the most convenient and widely used.

Transwell 是一类有通透性的杯状的装置,类似一种膜滤器(membrane filters),也可认为是一种有通透性的支架(permeable supports)。更精准地说,Transwell 应该是一种实验技术,这项技术的主要材料是 Transwell 小室(Transwell chamber or Transwell insert)。其外形为一个可放置在孔板里的小杯子,根据实验需要,可有不同选择。其关键部分都是一致的,那就是杯子底层是一张有通透性的膜,而杯子其余部分的材料与普通的孔板一样。这层膜带有微孔,孔径大小有 $0.1 \sim 12.0\ \mu m$,根据不同需要可用不同材料,一般常用的是聚碳酸酯膜(polycarbonate membrane)。将 Transwell 小室放入培养板中,小室内称上室,培养板内称下室,上室内盛装上层培养液,下室内盛装下层培养液,上下层培养液以聚碳酸酯膜相隔。将细胞种在上室内,由于聚碳酸酯膜有通透性,下层培养液中的成分可以影响到上室内的细胞,从而可以研究下层培养液中的成分对细胞生长、运动等的影响。应用不同孔径和经过不同处理的聚碳酸酯膜,就可以进行共培养、细胞趋化、细胞迁移和细胞侵袭等多种方面的研究。

The Transwell invasion assay is a simple and versatile tool to study cell invasion. This assay is based on two medium-containing chambers, with one (top) chamber inserted into the second (bottom) chamber. The floor of the top chamber comprises a porous membrane that has been coated with a layer of extracellular matrix (ECM). The ECM layer occludes the membrane pores and thereby prevents the movement of normal cells from the top to the bottom chamber. By contrast, invasive cells degrade the EMC and move through the ECM layer into the bottom chamber. Invasive cells that pass through the membrane pores adhere to the bottom of the filter and can be stained and counted using a microscope. This assay can be adapted for the study of different cell lines by varying pores sizes and the composition of the ECM. This assay has been successfully used to study cellular invasion of many types of medically important cells, including human trophoblasts, melanomas and colon cancer cells.

(一) 仪器与试剂　Required equipment and reagents

24 孔细胞培养板、Transwell 小室、无血清培养基、5%～10% FBS 的培养基、0.1%结晶紫、细胞培养箱。

24-well cell culture plates, Transwell chamber, serum-free medium, culture medium (5%～10% FBS), 0.1% crystal violet, cell culture incubator.

(二) 操作步骤　Protocols

1. 有基质胶的 Transwell 小室制备　Preparation of transwell chamber with matrigel

将小室放入 24 孔细胞培养板中,在上室加入 300 μl 预温的无血清培养基,室温下静置 15～30 min,吸去培养液。

Put the chamber into the 24-well plate, add 300 μl pre-warmed serum-free medium to the upper chamber for 15 to 30 minutes at room temperature. Suck out the medium.

2. 制备细胞悬液　Preparation of cell suspension

(1) 制备细胞悬液前可先以无血清培养基洗涤细胞。

Wash the cells with serum-free medium.

(2) 消化细胞:终止消化后离心弃去培养液,用 PBS 洗 2 遍,用含 1% BSA 的无血清培养基重悬。调整细胞密度至 $(1 \sim 10) \times 10^5$ 个/ml。

Digest the cells and discard the culture solution after the digestion, wash the cells with

PBS twice. Adjust the cell density to 1×10^5 to 10×10^5 cells/ml with the serum-free medium(1% BSA).

3. 接种细胞　Seeding cells

(1) 取细胞悬液 200 μl 加入 Transwell 小室。

Add 200 μl cell suspension per well to the Transwell chamber.

(2) 24 孔板下室加入 500 μl 含 FBS(5%~10%)或趋化因子的培养基,避免出现气泡。

Add 500 μl of culture medium (5% to 10% FBS) to the lower chamber of the 24-well plate. Avoid air bubbles.

4. 培养细胞　Cell culture

常规培养 12~48 h(主要依细胞侵袭能力而定)。时间点的选择除了要考虑到细胞侵袭力外,处理因子对细胞数目的影响也不可忽视。

Return cells to the incubator for 12 to 48 h (depending on the ability of the cell invasion).

5. 结果统计　Results analysis

(1) 直接计数法 Direct counting:"贴壁"细胞数:这里所谓的"贴壁"是指细胞穿过膜后,可以附着在膜的下室侧而不会掉到下室里面去。通过细胞染色,可在镜下计数细胞。

"Adherent" cell number: the "adherent" refers to the cells passing through the membrane, which can attach to the lower side of the membrane, not fall into the lower chamber. Cells can be counted under the microscope by cell staining.

1) 用棉签擦去基质胶和上室内的细胞。

Use cotton swab to wipe off the basic glue and cells in the upper chamber.

2) 用 0.1% 结晶紫染色。

Stain cells with 0.1% crystal violet.

3) 显微镜下随机选取 5 个视野计数细胞个数。

Randomly select five visual fields to count the number of cells under microscope.

"非贴壁"细胞计数:由于某些细胞自身的原因或某些膜的关系,有时细胞在穿过膜后不能附着在膜上,而是掉进下室。可以收集下层培养液,用流式细胞仪计数细胞量,也可用细胞计数的方法直接在镜下计数。

For the "non-adherent" cell, choose the flow cytometry to detect the cell quantity of the subculture medium. The number of cells can also be counted directly under microscope.

(2) 间接计数法 indirect counting:间接计数法主要用于穿过细胞过多,而无法通过计数获得准确的细胞数所采用的方法,与常用的 MTT 实验是同样的原理。

If too many cells pass through, the exact number of cells cannot be counted. The indirect counting will be used,which principle is the same as MTT assay.

1) 用棉签擦去基质胶和上室内的细胞。

Wipe off the basic glue and the cells in the upper chamber with cotton swab.

2) 24 孔培养板中加入 500 μl 含 0.5 mg/ml MTT 的完全培养基,将小室置于其中,使膜浸没在培养基中,37℃ 4 h 后取出。

Add 500 μl full medium (containing 0.5 mg/ml MTT) per well, immerse the chamber membrane in the medium. Incubate 4 hours at 37℃.

3) 24 孔培养板中加入 500 μl DMSO,将小室置于其中,使膜浸没在 DMSO 中,振荡 10 min,使甲臢充分溶解。取出小室,24 孔板于酶标仪上测 OD 值。

Add 500 μl DMSO, immerse the membrane in DMSO and oscillate for 10 minutes. Take out the chamber and measure the OD value.

(三)注意事项 Notes

(1) 上层培养液:无血清培养基,为维持渗透压,需加入 0.05%～0.2% BSA;下层培养液:下层常用含 5%～10% FBS 的培养基,具体浓度根据细胞侵袭力而定,侵袭力弱的细胞可适当提高 FBS 浓度;膜的下室面可涂上纤维粘连蛋白(fibronectin,FN),也可用胶原(collagen)或明胶(gelatin)。

Upper culture medium: serum-free medium. To maintain osmotic pressure, add 0.05% to 0.2% BSA. Lower medium: the medium containing 5% to 10% FBS.

(2) 常用的染色方法有结晶紫染色、台盼蓝染色、Giemsa 染色、苏木精染色、伊红染色等。

The usual staining methods include crystal violet staining, trypan blue staining, Giemsa staining, hematoxylin staining, and eosin staining.

(3) 使用正置显微镜进行观察和拍照时,可把 Transwell 小室反过来底朝上就可清楚看到小室底膜上下室侧附着的细胞。也可用手术刀将膜切下染色后,再贴在玻片上,滴二甲苯,盖上盖玻片,可以长期保存。

The Transwell chamber can be observed and photographed under a microscope, and the fine attachment of the chamber below and below the ependymal membrane could be clearly seen on the upside of the bottom of the chamber. The membrane can also be cut with scalpel and stain, and then put it on the slide. Drop xylene on the membrane, and cover with a overslip for long-term storage.

（于文静）

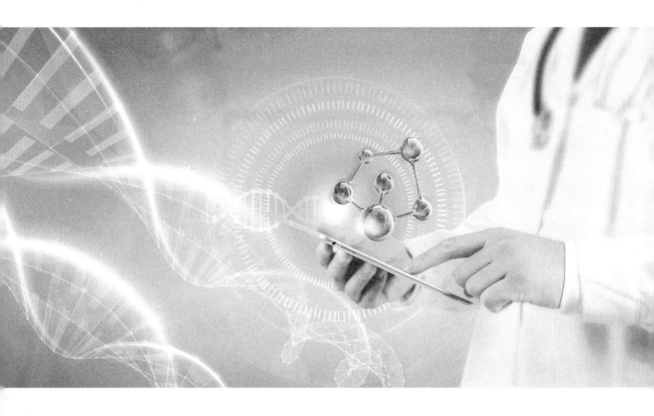

第二篇
细胞的遗传物质
Genetic material of cells

第六章　细胞内核酸的提取
Nucleic acid extraction

人类基因组计划的完成以及后基因组学研究的不断深入,标志着现代医学的发展已逐步进入"基因组医学"的时代。疾病分子机制的研究也将为包括疾病的分子诊断、分子治疗在内的"分子医学"的发展提供动力。

核酸是遗传信息以及基因表达的物质基础,是重要的生物信息分子,也是分子生物学研究的主要对象。核酸与生命的正常活动,如种族遗传、生长等有密切联系;与生命的异常活动,如肿瘤的发生、放射损伤以及抗癌、抗病毒药物的作用机制等也有密切的关系。因此,核酸是现代生命科学体系中重点研究的课题之一。核酸分为 DNA 和 RNA 两大类。核酸的提取是分子生物学实验技术中基本的操作之一。

The sequencing of the human genome in 2003, subsequent development of rapid and inexpensive DNA sequencing methods, and the growing sophistication of post-genomics analysis was established "genomic medicine" as a cutting-edge field of modern medicine. The isolation of DNA and RNA from human tissues and cell lines is an essential step in many medical research projects and for applying the techniques and insights of genomic medicine to the diagnosis, treatment and prevention of disease in individual patients.

第一节 ◉ 真核细胞基因组 DNA 的提取
Genomic DNA extraction from eukaryotic cells

DNA 主要在细胞核内,核外也有少量称为核外基因的线粒体 DNA 等。真核细胞的 DNA 分子比原核生物的 DNA 分子大得多,并且以核蛋白体形式存在于细胞中。真核细胞基因组 DNA 提取主要包括裂解和纯化两大步骤。裂解是使样品中的核酸游离在裂解体系中的过程,纯化则是去除体系中的其他成分,如蛋白质、多糖、脂类及其他不需要的核酸(RNA)等生物大分子的过程。

Genomic DNA is located primarily within the cellular nucleus, with addition small amounts located within mitochondria. DNA extraction from eukaryotic cells begins with cell lysis and release from the cell nucleus. DNA purification involves the separation of DNA from other cellular components, including proteins, polysaccharides, lipids and RNA.

一、裂解　Lysis

细胞破碎的物理方式常为超声波、组织匀浆、液氮破碎以及包埋组织的超薄切片等。而为了获得大量完整的 DNA,一般采用裂解液等温和的方法破碎细胞。

裂解液一般都含有去污剂(如 SDS、Triton X‑100、NP‑40、Tween 20 等)和盐(如 Tris、EDTA、NaCl 等)。去污剂的作用是通过使蛋白质变性,破坏膜结构及去除与核酸相连接的蛋白质,从而实现核酸游离在裂解体系中。盐的作用,一方面提供一个合适的裂解环境(如 Tris);另一方面,可抑制核酸酶在裂解过程中对核酸的破坏(如 EDTA)、维持核酸结构的稳定(如 NaCl)。裂解体系中还可以加入蛋白酶,利用蛋白酶将蛋白质消化成小的片段,促进核酸与蛋白质的分离,便于后面的纯化操作以及获得更纯的核酸。

To obtain large amounts of genomic DNA, cells are usually broken up by isothermal lysis in buffers containing detergents, such as SDS, Triton X‑100, or NP‑40, Tween 20, and salts, such as Tris‑HCL, sodium EDTA, and NaCl. Proteases are also often added digest proteins into smaller fragments to promote the separation of nucleic acids from proteins.

二、纯化　Purification

根据 DNA 本身的特征使用不同方法进行核酸提纯。

Different types of DNA purification methods are available for different types of DNA.

三、组织或培养细胞的 DNA 提取　DNA extracted from tissue and cultured cells

(一)仪器与试剂　Required equipment and reagents

消化液、25 mmol/L EDTA (pH 8.0)、PBS、TES 饱和酚、氯仿、异戊醇、95%乙醇溶液、70%乙醇溶液、TE 缓冲液、0.1% SDS、1 μg/ml RNA 酶、培养皿、培养瓶、微量离心管、离心机、液氮罐和恒温培养箱。

Digestive solution, 25 mmol/L EDTA (pH 8.0), PBS, TES saturated phenol, chloroform, isoamyl ethanol, 95% ethanol solution, 70% ethanol solution, TE buffer, 0.1% SDS, 1 μg/ml RNA enzyme, petri dishes, culture flasks, microcentrifuge tubes, centrifuge, liquid nitrogen tank, constant temperature incubator.

(二)主要步骤　Protocols

(1) 如果材料为组织块,可将组织块(200~1 000 mg)剪碎后,置入液氮中。随后用冰冷的组织捣碎器捣碎,每 100 mg 组织加入 1.2 ml 消化液。

If the material is tissue block: cut the tissue block (200~1 000 mg), put into liquid nitrogen, and add 1.2 ml of digestive solution per 100 mg tissue.

(2) 如果材料是悬浮细胞,收集细胞于微量离心管中,500×g 离心 5 min;如果材料是贴壁细胞,弃上清液后,胰蛋白酶消化收集细胞,500×g 离心 5 min。随后用冷 PBS 洗涤细胞,500×g 离心 5 min,弃上清液。PBS 重复洗涤一次,离心弃上清液,并用 1 倍体积的消化液重悬细胞。

If the material is suspended cells: harvest cells, transfer cells in a microcentrifuge tube, centrifuge at $500 \times g$ for 5 min, discard the supernatant. If the material is adherent cells: discard the supernatant, harvest cells by trypsinization, centrifuge at $500 \times g$ for 5 min, discard the supernatant. Wash cells with cold PBS, centrifuge at $500 \times g$ for 5 min, discard the supernatant. Repeat again, and suspend cells with double volume of digestive solution.

（3）将组织或细胞混悬液移入离心管中,50℃消化 12～18 h。

Transfer tissue or cell suspension into a centrifuge tube, digest at 50℃ for 12 to 18 h.

（4）冷却至 4℃,加等体积 15 mol/L TES 饱和酚。

Add equal volume of 15 mol/L TES saturated phenol to tissue or cell suspension at 4℃.

（5）震荡 1 min,使水相和酚层充分混匀。

Vortex 1 minute to make the water phase and the phenol layer fully mixed.

（6）4℃,5 000～8 000 r/min 离心 15～20 min。此时 DNA 溶液在上层,酚位于下层,中间是变性蛋白层。

Centrifuge at 5 000 to 8 000 r/min at 4℃ for 15 to 20 minutes. Then DNA solution is in the upper layer, phenol is in the lower layer, and denatured protein layer is in the middle.

（7）用吸管小心吸取上层粘稠的 DNA 溶液,移至另一离心管（管 1）。

Carefully transfer the viscous solution from the upper layer to another centrifuge tube (TUBE 1).

（8）DNA 溶液再加等体积 15 mol/L TES 饱和酚抽提一次,重复步骤 5、6、7,并将上层溶液吸至另一离心管（管 2）。

Add equal volume of 15 mol/L TES saturated phenol to TUBE 1, repeat step5, 6 and 7, and transfer the DNA solution to a new centrifuge tube (TUBE 2).

（9）向管 2 中加等体积氯仿/异戊醇,震荡 1 min,4℃,5 000～8 000 r/min 离心 15～20 min。

Add equal volume of chloroform/isoamyl ethanol solution to TUBE 2, vortex for 1 min. Centrifuge at 5 000 to 8 000 r/min at 4℃ for 15 to 20 minutes.

（10）尽可能多地吸取上层溶液,移至另一离心管（管 3）。

Transfer as much of the top aqueous solution as possible to a new centrifuge tube (TUBE 3). Avoid picking up any of the chloroform/isoamyl ethanol phase.

（11）重复步骤 9,并吸取上层溶液至新的离心管（管 4）,置于冰上。

Repeat step 9, and transfer the top solution to a new centrifuge tube (TUBE 4). Put TUBE 4 on ice.

（12）加 2.5 倍体积 95% 冷乙醇,充分混匀。

Add 2.5 times volume of 95% cold ethanol and mix well.

（13）加入 600 μl 75% 冷乙醇清洗。4℃,12 000 r/min 离心 15 min,弃上清液。

Wash by adding 600 μl of 75% cold ethanol. Centrifuge at 12 000 r/min at 4℃ for 15 minutes, discard supernatant carefully without disturbing the pellet.

（14）重复步骤 13 两次。

Repeat step 13 twice.

（15）室温干燥 3 min。

Air dry for 3 minutes.

（16）加适量 TE 溶液溶解 DNA。

Re-suspend pellet in appropriate volume of TE buffer.

（三）结果鉴定 Quantitative and qualitative assessment of DNA

（1）紫外分光光度计检测：可检测 DNA 的纯度和含量。一般而言核酸在 260 nm 时吸光度最大，而蛋白质在 280 nm 时吸光度最大。紫外分光光度计测定 260、280 nm 的 OD 值，计算 OD_{260}/OD_{280} 比值，比值在 1.8 左右，说明 DNA 纯度可。在 260 nm 处，1 OD 双链 DNA 的浓度为 50 μg/ml，据此可计算 DNA 的浓度（μg/ml）＝50×（OD_{260}）×稀释倍数。

Ultraviolet spectrophotometer detection: To measure DNA concentration and purity. Nucleic acids absorb UV light most strongly at 260 nm, while proteins absorb most strongly at 280 nm. The ratio of absorbance at 260 nm (OD_{260}) and 280 nm (OD_{280}) is used to assess the purify of DNA. The ratio of 1.8 is generally accepted as "pure" for DNA. At 260 nm, the concentration of 1 OD double-stranded DNA is 50 μg/ml, so double-stranded DNA concentration (μg/ml)＝50 μg/ml×OD_{260}×dilution factor.

（2）电泳检测：可检测核酸的完整性和大小。取 2 μl DNA 溶解液与适量上样缓冲液混合后，经 1% 琼脂糖凝胶电泳。电泳结束后紫外光下观察，拍照。如果观察到一条清晰的电泳带，无明显的拖尾，说明 DNA 完整性好。

Electrophoretic detection: To detect the integrity and size of nucleic acid. Mix 2 μl DNA solution with an appropriate sample buffer, and perform 1% agarose gel electrophoresis. After the electrophoresis, observe and photograph the DNA under ultraviolet light. If a clear electrophoretic band is observed and no obvious tail is observed, the DNA integrity is good.

（四）附录 Appendix

消化液：100 mmol/L NaCl、10 mmol/L Tris－HCl（pH 8.0）、25 mmol/L EDTA、0.5% SDS 和 0.1 mg/ml 蛋白酶 K。

Digestive solution: 100 mmol/L NaCl, 10 mmol/L Tris－HCl（pH 8.0），25 mmol/L EDTA, 0.5% SDS and 0.1 mg/ml protease K.

第二节 ◉ 真核细胞总 RNA 的提取和反转录
Total RNA isolation and reverse transcription

RNA 是基因表达产物，由以下几类分子组成，rRNA（占细胞总 RNA 的 80%～85%）、tRNA 和核内小分子 RNA（占 10%～15%）、mRNA（占 1%～5%）。其中 mRNA 是分子生物学的主要研究对象,分离制备 mRNA 是克隆基因,分析基因表达以及建立 cDNA 文库的首要步骤。

真核细胞总 RNA 分离提取的目的是要获得高纯度的具有充分长度的 RNA 分子,包括 RNA 的纯度和完整性。RNA 分离的关键是尽量减少 RNA 酶(RNases)的污染。RNA 酶活性非常稳定,分布广泛,除细胞内源性的 RNA 酶外,环境中也存在 RNA 酶。因此,在提取 RNA 时,应尽量创造一个无 RNA 酶的环境,包括去除外源性 RNA 酶的污染和抑制内源性 RNA 酶活性。主要是采用 RNA 酶的阻抑蛋白 RNasin 和强力的蛋白变性剂盐酸胍或异硫氰酸胍抑制内源性 RNA 酶,采用焦碳酸二乙酯(diethyl pyrocarbonate,DEPC)去除外源性 RNA 酶。

RNA is the direct product of gene expression and an important target for basic and medical research. Isolation of RNA is the important step for cloning genes, analyzing gene expression and establishing cellular and tissue-based expression libraries. These applications usually require intact RNA of high purity. Because RNA is especially sensitive to degradation by cellular RNases, care must be taken to prevent exposure to these enzymes during isolation.

一、RNA 提取的关键 The key to RNA extraction

真核细胞 RNA 的提取过程有 4 个关键点:①样品(细胞或组织)的有效破碎;②有效地使核蛋白复合体变性;③对内源 RNA 酶的有效抑制;④有效地将 RNA 从 DNA 和蛋白混合物中分离;其中最关键的是抑制 RNA 酶的活性。提取的 RNA 可以用于核酸杂交、cDNA 合成以及体外翻译等。

There are four key points during RNA extraction from eukaryotic cells: ①effective fragmentation of samples (cells or tissues); ② effective denaturation of nucleoprotein complexes; ③effective inhibition of endogenous RNases; ④effective isolation of RNA from DNA and protein mixtures; and the most critical one is inhibition of RNases activity.

二、组织 RNA 的提取 RNA extracted from tissue

(一)仪器与试剂 Required equipments and reagents

TRIzol、氯仿、75%乙醇、异丙醇、DEPC 水、变性胶缓冲液、37%甲醛、3%过氧化氢、甲酰胺、RNA 上样缓冲液、无核酸酶离心管、无核酸酶枪头、组织匀浆器和离心机。

TRIzol, chloroform, 75% ethanol, isopropanol, DEPC-treated water, denaturing gel buffer, 37% formaldehyde, 3% hydrogen peroxide, formamide, RNA sample loading buffer, nuclease-free centrifuge tubes, nuclease-free tips, tissue homogenizer, centrifuge.

(二)操作步骤 Protocols

(1) 取 50~100 mg 组织匀浆后移入离心管,加入 0.8 ml TRIzol,冰上静置 5 min。

Homogenize 50 to 100 mg tissue with tissue homogenizer, and transfer to a centrifuge tube. Add 0.8 ml TRIzol in the tube, and put on ice for 5 minutes.

(2) 加 0.2 ml 氯仿,充分震荡混匀,静置 3 min,4℃,12 000×g 离心 15 min。

Add 0.2 ml chloroform, vortex and mix, stand for 3 minutes. Centrifuge at 12 000×g

at 4℃ for 15 minutes.

（3）取上清液，加入 0.5 ml 异丙醇，颠倒混匀 3～4 次。－20℃ 静置 2 h，4℃，12 000×g 离心 10 min。

Transfer the supernatant to a new centrifuge tube，add 0.5 ml isopropanol and invert tube 3 to 4 times．Stand at － 20℃ for 2 hours．Centrifuge at 12 000 × g at 4℃ for 10 minutes．

（4）弃上清液，取沉淀物，加入 1 ml 75% 乙醇溶液，漂洗沉淀物，4℃，7 500×g 离心 5 min。

Discard the supernatant，take the pellet，add 1 ml 75% ethanol solution to wash the pellet．Centrifuged at 7 500×g at 4℃ for 5 minutes．

（5）弃上清液，干燥沉淀物 10 min。

Discard the supernatant，air dry the RNA pellet for 10 minutes．

（6）加 40 μl DEPC 水，充分溶解 RNA 沉淀。

Add 40 μl DEPC-treated water to resuspend the RNA pellet．

（三）结果鉴定　Result identification

（1）紫外分光光度计检测：紫外分光光度计测定 260、280 nm 的 OD 值，计算 OD_{260}/OD_{280} 比值，比值在 2.0 左右，说明 RNA 纯度可。在 260 nm 处，1 OD RNA 的浓度为 40 μg/ml，据此可计算 RNA 的浓度（μg/ml）＝40 μg/ml×（OD_{260}）×稀释倍数。

Ultraviolet spectrophotometer detection：To measure RNA concentration and purity．The ratio of absorbance at 260 nm （OD_{260}） and 280 nm （OD_{280}） is used to assess the purify of RNA．The ratio of 2.0 is generally accepted as "pure" for RNA．At 260 nm，the concentration of 1 OD RNA is 40 μg/ml，so double-stranded DNA concentration （μg/ml）＝40 μg/ml×OD_{260}×dilution factor．

（2）电泳检测：1% 甲醛变性胶电泳观察 RNA 质量。如果观察到清晰的 18S、28S RNA 电泳带，无大量小分子 RNA，说明 RNA 无明显降解，样品 －70℃ 保存备用。

Electrophoretic detection：To detect the quality of RNA by 1% formaldehyde denaturing gel electrophoresis．If clear 18S，28S RNA electrophoresis bands are observed without large number of small RNAs，indicate that there is no obvious degradation of RNA．Store the sample at －70℃．

三、反转录（AMV 反转录酶法）　Reverse transcription （AMV reverse transcriptase）

（一）仪器与试剂　Required equipments and reagents

DEPC 水、引物、AMV 反转录酶、无核酸酶离心管、无核酸酶枪头、离心机。

DEPC-treated water，primer，AMV Reverse Transcriptase，nuclease-free centrifuge tubes，nuclease-free tips，centrifuge．

（二）操作步骤　Protocols

（1）无核酸酶离心管内加入 4.5 μl DEPC 水，1 μl 引物，1 μl 模板 RNA，混匀。

Mix 4.5 μl DEPC-treated water，1 μl primer and 1 μl template RNA in a nuclease-free centrifuge tube.

（2）瞬时离心，100℃放置 1 min。

Centrifuge slightly and heat to 100℃ for 1 minutes.

（3）加入 0.5 μl dNTP，2 μl 5×Buffer，1 μl AMV 反转录酶。

Add 0.5 μl dNTP，2 μl 5×Buffer，1 μl AMV reverse transcriptase.

（4）瞬时离心，42℃孵育 90 min。

Slightly centrifuge，incubate at 42℃ for 90 minutes.

（5）100℃孵育 3 min 灭活 AMV 反转录酶。

Incubate at 100℃ for 3 minutes to inactivate AMV Reverse Transcriptase.

（6）−20℃ 保存。

Store the sample at −20℃.

四、注意事项　Notes

（1）所用试剂均用 DEPC 水配制。

Prepare all the reagents with DEPC-treated water.

（2）实验操作过程中要戴一次性手套，以避免 RNA 酶污染。

Wear gloves during the experiment to avoid RNase contamination.

第三节 ◎ 质粒 DNA 的提取
Plasmid DNA isolation

细菌质粒是一类大小 1～200 kb 的双链共价闭合环状 DNA，存在于细胞质中、独立于细胞染色体之外的可自主复制的遗传成份。通常情况下可持续稳定地处于染色体外的游离状态，但在一定条件下也会可逆地整合到寄主染色体上，随着染色体的复制而复制，并通过细胞分裂传递到后代。质粒是目前最常用的基因克隆的载体分子之一，获得大量纯化的质粒 DNA 是基因克隆的前提条件。

Bacterial plasmids comprise covalently closed，circular DNA molecules containing 1 to 200 kilo base（kb）pairs. Bacterial plasmids are self-replicating units that function independently of bacterial genomic DNA. Bacterial plasmids are widely used for cloning of eukaryotic genes and for construction of eukaryotic gene expression libraries. They have also been extensively engineered for use in functional studies of eukaryotic cells，for example as molecular reporters for eukaryotic gene expression. Obtaining large amounts of purified plasmid DNA from bacteria is an important first step in using plasmids in basic medical research.

一、碱裂解法提取质粒 DNA 的原理　Principle of plasmid DNA isolation by alkaline lysis method

碱裂解法是一种应用最为广泛的制备质粒 DNA 的方法，其基本原理为：共价闭合环状

DNA 与线性 DNA 的拓扑学性质不同。在 pH 12～12.5 时,线性 DNA 会完全变性,而共价闭合环状 DNA 只是氢键断裂,经酸中和后,共价闭合环状 DNA 可迅速精准确地复性。而线性 DNA 不能精准确地复性,只能聚合成网状结构,离心后与变性的蛋白质、RNA 一起沉淀下来。上清液中的质粒 DNA 可用乙醇沉淀出来。

Alkaline lysis method is one of the most widely used methods for isolating plasmid DNA. It is based on the observation that covalently closed circular DNA has different properties from linear DNA. At pH 12 to 12.5, linear DNA will be completely denatured into separate DNA strands. By contrast, covalently closed cyclic DNA undergoes disruption of hydrogen between its components the nucleic acid bases, but remains double-stranded. Following neutralization, the covalently closed plasmid DNA rapidly and accurately renatures. Linear DNA, on the other hand, cannot accurately renature and instead becomes aggregated into an extensive network that can be precipitated along with denatured proteins and RNA by centrifugation. Plasmid DNA that remains in supernatant can be precipitated by addition of ethanol.

二、碱裂解法提取质粒 DNA　Plasmid DNA isolation by alkaline lysis method

(一)仪器与试剂　Required equipment and reagents

溶液 Ⅰ、溶液 Ⅱ、pH 4.8 的醋酸钾(KAc)缓冲液、TE 缓冲液、苯酚/氯仿/异戊醇(25:24:1)、无水乙醇、70%乙醇、TBE 缓冲液、10 mg/ml 溴化乙锭(ethidium bromide, EB)、琼脂糖、10 mg/ml 核糖核酸酶 A(RNase A)、6×上样缓冲液、离心机、电泳仪、水平式电泳槽。

Solution Ⅰ, solution Ⅱ, potassium acetate (KAc) buffer (pH 4.8), TE buffer, phenol/chloroform/isoamyl ethanol (25:24:1), absolute ethanol, 70% ethanol, TBE buffer, 10 mg/ml ethidium bromide (EB), agarose, 10 mg/ml RNase A, 6 × loading buffer, centrifuge, electrophoresis apparatus, horizontal electrophoresis tank.

(二)操作步骤　Protocols

(1)挑取 LB 固体培养基上生长的大肠杆菌单菌落,接种于 2.0 ml LB(含相应抗生素)液体培养基中,37℃振荡培养过夜。

Select single colonies of Escherichia coli (E. coli) grown on LB solid medium and inoculate it into 2.0 ml LB liquid medium containing antibiotics. Culture the colonies overnight at 37℃.

(2)取 1.5 ml 培养物转移入微量离心管中,室温 8 000×g 离心 1 min,弃上清液,将离心管倒置,使液体尽可能流尽。

Transfer 1.5 ml of cultures to a centrifuge tube, Centrifuge at 8 000×g for 1 minutes at room temperature, discarded the supernatant. Invert the centrifuge tube to make the liquid as exhausted as possible.

(3)将细菌沉淀重悬于 100 μl 预冷的溶液 Ⅰ 中,剧烈振荡。

Resuspend the pellet in 100 μl pre-cooled solution Ⅰ and vortex.

(4)加 200 μl 新鲜配制的溶液 Ⅱ 于离心管中,颠倒数次混匀(不要剧烈振荡),并将离心管放置于冰上 2～3 min,使细胞膜充分裂解。

Add 200 μl fresh solution Ⅱ to the centrifuge tube, gently invert several times, and place on ice for 2 to 3 minutes to break up the cell membrane.

（5）加入 150 μl 预冷的醋酸钾(KAc)缓冲液,将离心管温和颠倒数次混匀,见白色絮状沉淀,可在冰上放置 3～5 min。

Add 150 μl pre-cooled potassium acetate buffer, gently invert several times, place on ice for 3 to 5 minutes.

（6）加入 450 μl 的苯酚/氯仿/异戊醇混合液,振荡混匀,4℃，12 000×g 离心 10 min。

Add 450 μl of the mixture of phenol/chloroform/isoamyl ethanol, mix and centrifuge at 12 000×g for 10 minutes at 4℃.

（7）小心移出上清液至另一微量离心管中,加入 2.5 倍体积预冷的无水乙醇,混匀,室温放置 2～5 min,4℃，12 000×g 离心 15 min。

Remove the supernatant carefully and place it in another centrifuge tube. Add 2.5 times volume of pre-cooled anhydrous ethanol and mix it. Place the centrifuge tube at room temperature for 2 to 5 minutes and centrifuge at 12 000×g for 15 minutes at 4℃.

（8）加入 1 ml 预冷的 70%乙醇洗涤沉淀 2 次,4℃，8 000×g 离心 7 min,弃上清液,将沉淀物在室温下晾干。

Wash the pellet twice with 1 ml of pre-cooled 70% ethanol, centrifuge at 8 000×g for 7 min at 4℃, discard supernatant, and air dry at room temperature.

（9）将沉淀物溶于 20 μl TE(含 RNase A 20 μg/ml),－20℃ 保存备用。

Dissolve the pellet in 20 μl TE (containing RNase A 20 μg/ml), store at －20℃.

（三）结果鉴定 Result identification

1%琼脂糖凝胶电泳检测,方法同核酸 DNA 的鉴定。

Electrophoretic detection: use 1% agarose gel electrophoresis. The same methods as identifying genomic DNA.

（四）附录 Appendix

（1）溶液 Ⅰ :50 mmol 葡萄糖,25 mmol Tris－HCl(pH 8.0),10 mmol EDTA(pH 8.0)。

Solution Ⅰ :50 mmol glucose,25 mmol Tris－HCl (pH 8.0),10 mmol EDTA (pH 8.0).

（2）溶液Ⅱ:0.2 mol NaOH,1% SDS。

Solution Ⅱ:0.2 mol NaOH,1% SDS.

第四节 ◎ 线粒体 DNA 的提取
Mitochondrial DNA isolation

线粒体 DNA(mitochondrial DNA,mtDNA)是染色体遗传物质,哺乳类动物的线粒体 DNA 为共价闭合环状的双链 DNA。它变异快、结构相对简单,经母系遗传,对真核生物基因组的结构、复制、转录、调控机制等方面都起着重要作用。近年来,被广泛用于近缘种间或种内种群间亲缘关系的研究。

线粒体 DNA 最早是用氯化铯梯度离心方法获得。该法提取的线粒体 DNA 纯度高，但所需仪器设备昂贵，实验周期长，限制其在群体遗传研究中的应用。继而出现了 Triton 法、碱变性法与改进高盐沉淀法等线粒体 DNA 的提取方法。

Mammalian mitochondrial DNA comprises covalently closed, circular DNA molecules similar to bacterial plasmids. Isolation of mitochondrial DNA is important for diagnosis of mitochondrial genetic disorders and for basic research on the underlying molecular mechanisms of those disorders. Mitochondrial DNA has traditionally been isolated using cesium chloride gradient centrifugation. The purity of mitochondrial DNA extracted by this method is high, but the equipment required is expensive and isolation process time-consuming. Currently, methods employing Triton-based cellular lysis, followed by alkaline denaturation method and high salt precipitation are widely used for the isolation of mitochondrial DNA.

一、碱变性法提取线粒体 DNA 的原理 Principle of mitochondrial DNA isolation by alkaline lysis method

线粒体 DNA 的结构与质粒 DNA 的结构相似，均为共价闭合环状的双链 DNA，实验原理与质粒 DNA 提取相同。

The experimental principles underlying this method are similar to those used for the isolation of plasmid DNA from bacteria.

二、碱变性法提取线粒体 DNA Mitochondrial DNA isolation by alkaline lysis method

（一）仪器与试剂 Required equipment and reagents

50 mmol/L 葡萄糖、10 mmol/L Na₂EDTA、25 mmol/L Tris－HCl (pH 8.0)、1％SDS、0.2 M NaOH、3 mol 醋酸钠(NaAc)(pH 4.8)、95％乙醇、75％乙醇、TE 缓冲液、匀浆器、高速离心机、离心管、吸管。

50 mmol/L glucose, 10 mmol/L Na₂EDTA, 25 mmol/L Tris－HCl (pH 8.0), 1％ SDS, 0.2 M NaOH, 3 mol NaAc (pH 4.8), 95％ ethanol, 75％ ethanol, TE buffer, homogenizer, centrifuge, centrifuge tube, pipette.

（二）操作步骤 Protocols

（1）取 50 mg 新鲜小鼠肝组织，用匀浆器匀浆，随即 4℃，1 000×g 离心 3 min，弃沉淀物。

Homogenize 50 mg fresh liver tissue of mice by homogenizer, centrifuge at 1 000×g for 3 minutes at 4℃, discard the pellet.

（2）转移上清液至新的离心管，4℃，12 000×g 离心 10 min。

Transfer the supernatant to a new centrifuge tube, and centrifuge at 12 000×g for 10 minutes at 4℃.

（3）弃上清液，将沉淀物溶于 100 μl 溶液Ⅰ中，充分混匀。

Discard the supernatant and dissolve the pellet with 100 μl solution Ⅰ and mix.

（4）加 200 μl 新鲜配制的溶液Ⅱ，轻轻摇匀，冰浴 5 min。

Add 200 μl solution Ⅱ, gently shake, and put on ice for 5 minutes.

（5）加 150 μl 3 mol/L NaAc（pH 4.8)溶液，轻轻摇匀，冰浴 5 min。4℃，12 000×g 离心 10 min。

Add 150 μl of 3 mol/L NaAc（pH 4.8），gently shake, put on ice for 5 minutes. Centrifuge at 12 000×g for 10 minutes at 4℃.

（6）取上清液加等体积酚、氯仿、异戊醇混合液(体积比为 25：24：1)，10 000×g 离心 5 min。

Transfer the supernatant to a new centrifuge tube, and add the equal volume of a mixture solution（phenol, chloroform and isoamyl ethanol 25：24：1）. Centrifuge at 10 000×g for 5 minutes.

（7）取上清液加 2 倍体积 95％乙醇，室温静置 15 min，然后 12 000×g 离心 10 min。

Transfer the supernatant to a new centrifuge tube, add 2×volume of 95％ ethanol, centrifuge at 12 000×g for 15 minutes at room temperature.

（8）弃上清液，沉淀物用 75％乙醇洗涤 1 次，12 000×g 离心 5 min。

Discard the supernatant, wash the pellet with 75％ ethanol, and centrifuge at 12 000×g for 5 minutes.

（9）弃上清液，取沉淀物，干燥后即得线粒体 DNA。将其溶于适量的 TE 缓冲液中，－20℃ 保存。

Discard the supernatant, air dry at room temperature. Dissolve pellet with TE buffer, store at －20℃.

（三）实验结果鉴定　Identification of experimental results

用紫外分光光度仪测定，OD_{260}：OD_{280} 为 2.0 左右说明线粒体 DNA 较纯。

The ratio of OD_{260} and OD_{280} of 2.0 is generally accepted as "pure" for mtDNA.

（四）附录　Appendix

溶液Ⅰ：50 mmol/L 葡萄糖、10 mmol/L Na_2EDTA 和 25 mmol/L Tris－HCl（pH 8.0)。

Solution Ⅰ：50 mmol/L glucose, 10 mmol/L Na_2EDTA and 25 mmol/L Tris－HCl（pH 8.0).

（刘红英）

第七章　基因分析技术
Gene analysis techniques

　　基因是细胞内遗传物质的结构和功能单位。在世代交替过程中，基因保持其固有的分子组成并发挥其特定的生物学功能，最终表现为物种遗传性状的相对稳定。而基因突变将有可能导致遗传性状的改变，乃至疾病的发生。因此，针对基因的检测、分析是遗传病诊断、治疗和预防的关键。基因分析技术也是医学遗传学的重要内容。

　　Genes are the basic structural and functional units of heredity in living organisms. Genes encode information required to build and maintain cells and tissues and are the vehicles for transmitting that information to offspring. Mutations that change gene structure or regulation produce genetic variation that is evolutionarily essential for adaption and survival of species. Maladaptive mutation, however, are often the cause genetic disorders. The identification of genetic variants that contribute to human disorders is one of the major goals of current medical research. The hope is that this information will be useful for the identification of molecular targets for novel therapeutic drug and for early diagnosis and possible prevention of human disease.

第一节 ◉ 核酸杂交技术
Nucleic acid hybridization

　　核酸杂交(nucleic acid hybridization)是两条互补的核苷酸单链在特定的条件下退火形成异质双链的过程。核酸杂交是对核酸分子进行定性和定量检测的常用技术。自 Southern 于 1975 年创建了检测特异 DNA 的核酸杂交技术以来，在此基础上发展起来的其他核酸杂交技术已成为分子生物学的基本技术。

　　核酸杂交既可以是 DNA 与 DNA 链、RNA 与 RNA 链之间的杂交，又可以是 DNA 与 RNA 链之间的杂交；探针可以是基因克隆技术分离获得的、体外转录出的或是人工合成的核苷酸片段；探针的标记物可以是放射性同位素，或是一些非放射性物质如生物素、地高辛和荧光素等。

　　Nucleic acid hybridization is a process of annealing two complementary single DNA or RNA molecules under specific conditions to form double-stranded molecules. Hybridization is the basis for many commonly used methods for qualitative and quantitative detection of nucleic acids. Nucleic acid hybridization can occur between single strands of DNA or RNA and between DNA and RNA strands. Single-stranded DNA or RNA probes that allow the detection of specific DNA or RNA molecules can be obtained by DNA cloning, *in vitro* transcription of target DNA sequences or by chemical synthesis. Single-stranded DNA or RNA probes are often labeled with radioactive isotopes or non-radioactive molecules such as biotin, digoxygenin or fluorescein to allow their detection when used for quantification or localization of target DNA or RNA molecules.

一、Southern 杂交技术　Sourthern blotting

Southern 杂交技术是将凝胶电泳分离的酶切 DNA 片段通过印记法(imprinting)转移到硝酸纤维素膜上,检测标记过的探针是否与变性后的靶 DNA 发生杂交,而对靶 DNA 进行定性和定量的一项分子生物学技术,包括 DNA 印记转移和 DNA 杂交两部分内容。

Southern blotting (also named Southern hybridization) is a method for qualitative and quantitative analysis of target DNAs. In this method, DNA isolated from cells or tissues is digested with restriction enzyme to generate specific DNA fragments of varying lengths. These fragments are then resolved by slab gel electrophoresis (vertical dimension), alkaline denatured *in situ*, and blotted or electrophoretically transferred onto a nitrocellulose or nylon membrane (horizontal dimension). The spatially separated single-stranded DNA on the membrane is then exposed to a labeled single-stranded DNA or RNA probe that hybridizes to a specific target sequence. The location of DNA molecules on the membrane containing that sequence is revealed by exposing the membrane to photographic film (in the case or radioactively labeled probes), by secondary enzyme-medicated chemiluminescence or generation of an insoluble precipitate (in the case of biotin or digoxygenin-labeled probes) or by fluorescence under ultraviolet irradiation (in the case of fluorescein-labeled probes).

(一) Southern 杂交的流程　Southern blotting process

首先从组织或培养细胞中分离基因组 DNA,用一种或多种限制性核酸内切酶消化基因组 DNA,然后进行琼脂糖凝胶电泳分离,再对 DNA 进行原位碱变性后将 DNA 片段从胶上转移至固相支持物上(如尼龙膜或硝酸纤维素膜),用标记的 DNA 或 RNA 探针在膜上与转印后的 DNA 片段杂交,最后针对不同的探针标记物选择特定的检测方法如放射自显影法、比色法、荧光检测或化学发光检测来确定与探针互补的靶 DNA 的存在及位置,检验该核酸片段是否与已知的探针有同源序列(图 7-1)。

Genomic double-stranded DNA isolated from tissues or cultured cells is digested with one or more restriction endonucleases. The resulting DNA fragments are then separated according to size by electrophoresis in an agarose or polyacrylamide gel. After *in situ* alkaline denaturation, the single-stranded DNA fragments are transferred from gel to a nitrocellulose or nylon membrane and hybridized with labeled single stranded DNA or RNA probes. Finally, autoradiography and fluorescence detection is used to identify the DNA fragments containing sequences complimentary to the sequence in the probes (Fig. 7-1).

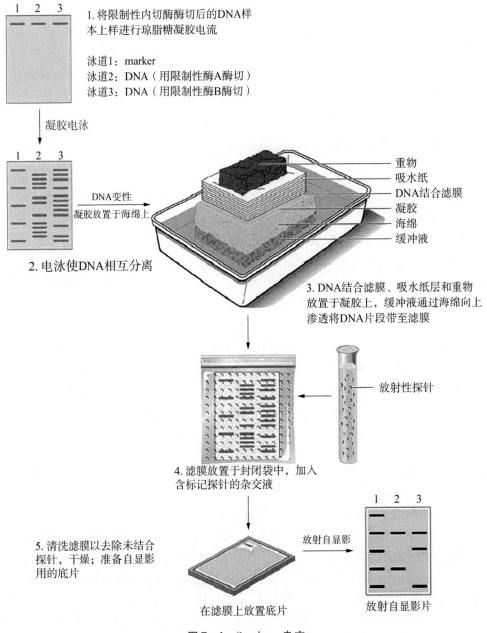

图 7 - 1　Southern 杂交

Fig. 7 - 1　Southern blotting

（二）注意事项　Notes

（1）选择限制性内切酶时应注意酶切位点的量要适当，一般消化前 DNA 的长度至少应为消化后长度的 3 倍。

To allow selection of appropriate restriction enzyme recognition sites，the length of DNA before digestion should be at least three times that after digestion.

（2）消化后的 DNA 上样前应于 56℃ 加热 3 min 以破坏粘性末端的连接。

The digested DNA should be heated for 3 minutes at 56℃ before loading onto the resolving gel to disrupt hybridization between extended 5′- or 3′ single-stranded "sticky" ends generated by some restriction enzymes.

（3）电泳后的凝胶放置不应超过 24 h,以免 DNA 条带扩散。

Gel should not be placed for more than 24 hours after electrophoresis，so as not to spread the DNA band.

（4）操作时,不能用手直接接触杂交膜,以免造成背景升高;膜一旦放置于凝胶上后,就不可再移动。

Hybridization membranes should always be handled with gloved hands.

（5）印记转移时,滤纸和杂交膜应完全湿润,并且凝胶、滤纸与杂交膜之间不能有气泡,以免影响转印效果。

When transferring DNA from the gel to the hybridization membrane，the filter paper and hybrid membrane should be completely moist，with no air bubbles between them.

二、Northern 杂交技术 Northern blotting

Northern 杂交（Northern blotting）技术是研究 RNA 印记转移和杂交的技术。与 Southern 杂交相类似,只是在上样前需要利用甲醛等变性剂使 RNA 变性。

Northern blotting（also named Northern hybridization）is a widely used method for detecting specific RNA molecules in extracts of cell or tissues.

（一）Northern 杂交的流程 Northern blotting process

Northern 杂交分析 RNA 的基本步骤是:首先从组织或细胞中分离总 RNA,用甲基氢氧化银、乙二醛或甲醛使 RNA 变性;然后通过无 EB 的琼脂糖凝胶变性电泳对 RNA 进行分离,电泳缓冲液常使用甲醛、甲酰胺等构成的 3-吗啉丙磺酸（MOPS）缓冲液;再将 RNA 转移到固相支持物上,如硝酸纤维素膜,并通过紫外线交联将其固定在支持物上（转移前需要将分子量标记物切胶、EB 染色、拍照）;再用含有标记物的探针与固定后的 RNA 杂交,洗脱除去非特异结合到固相支持物上的探针分子;最后对特异结合的探针分子的图象进行检测、捕获和分析。

Total RNA isolated from tissues or cells is denatured using methyl silver hydroxide, glyoxal or formaldehyde. The denatured RNA is resolved by gel electrophoresis under denaturing conditions before transfer to a nylon membrane and cross-linking to the membrane by exposure to ultraviolet light. Finally, specific binding of the labeled probe molecule is detected，captured and analyzed.

（二）注意事项 Notes

（1）所有操作均应避免 RNase 的污染。

Avoid RNase contamination.

（2）对小分子的 RNA 一般采用聚丙烯酰胺变性胶电泳。

Electrophoresis in polyacrylamide gel under denaturing conditions is generally used to resolve small RNA molecules.

（3）凝胶上的分子标记物泳道,应在电泳结束后,马上切下染色。用于杂交部分的 RNA 不能染色。因为胶中的 EB 会影响 RNA 与硝酸纤维素膜的结合。

After electrophoresis, cut and dye the gel Lane Marker (RNA Marker) immediately. Donot stain the RNA used for hybridization.

（4）印记转移时,滤纸转膜的缓冲液含有甲酰胺,可以降低 RNA 样本与探针的退火温度,减少高温环境对 RNA 降解。

In imprinting transfer, the buffer of filter paper transfer membrane contains formamide, which can reduce the annealing temperature of RNA samples and probes, and reduce the degradation of RNA in high temperature environment.

第二节 ◎ 聚合酶链反应
Polymerase chain reaction

聚合酶链反应(polymerase chain reaction,PCR)是一种体外核酸扩增技术,具有特异、敏感、产率高、快速、简便等突出优点。应用 PCR 技术可以在体外使特定的基因或 DNA 片段在很短的时间内扩增数十万至百万倍。扩增的片段可以直接通过电泳观察,并作进一步的分析。

Polymerase chain reaction (PCR) is a technique that is used to amplify a single or a few copies of DNA across several orders of magnitude, thus generating thousands to millions of copies of a particular DNA sequence.

一、实验原理 Experimental principle

PCR 是根据 DNA 变性复性的原理,通过特异性引物,完成特异片段扩增。具体流程包括:①引物设计,按照模板 DNA 的 5′和 3′端的碱基顺序各合成一段长 18～24 个碱基的寡核苷酸序列作为引物(primer);②混合反应体系,加入 4 种单核苷酸(dNTPs)、引物和耐热 DNA 聚合酶以及聚合酶缓冲液;③在 PCR 仪器上设置扩增程序:高温变性 DNA,低温使引物与模板 DNA 链复性结合(又称退火),在聚合酶的作用下,合适的温度延伸。执行 20～40 个循环程序后,就可以得到大量的 DNA 片段。理论上循环 20 周期可使 DNA 扩增 100 余万倍。

PCR, which is based on the principle of DNA denaturation and renaturation, uses specific primers to complete the amplification of specific fragments. The specific process is as follows. ①Design and synthesis of primer sequences of 18 to 24 bases on the 5′ and 3′ terminal base sequence of the template DNA; ②In the mixed reaction system, the four types of single nucleotides (dNTPs), primers, heat-resistant DNA polymerase, and polymerase buffer are added; ③The amplification program is set on the PCR instrument and includes (for each cycle) denaturation of DNA at high temperature, renaturation of the primers with the template DNA strands at low temperature (also known as annealing), and extension of DNA chains at medium temperature under the action of polymerase. A large number of DNA fragments can be obtained after the completion of 20 to 40 PCR cycles. In theory，a program of 20 cycles can amplify DNA more than one million times.

二、PCR 技术的分类及其应用范围 Classification and application of the PCR technology

（一）反转录 PCR Reverse transcription PCR

反转录 PCR(reverse transcription polymerase chain reaction，RT-PCR)是将 RNA 反转录成的 cDNA 为模板进行 PCR 扩增的一种技术。用于反转录的 RNA 模板要求完整，并且不含 DNA 和蛋白质等杂质。反转录引物可以采用 Oligo (dT)，随机引物或者基因特异性引物。

Reverse transcription polymerase chain reaction（RT-PCR）is a technique for PCR amplification using RNA as a template. The RNA template needs to be free of impurities. The reverse transcription primers can be oligo（dT），Random and sequence-specific primers.

（二）原位 PCR *In situ* PCR

原位 PCR 技术(*in situ* PCR)是将检测细胞内特定基因的原位杂交技术和 PCR 相结合的方法，是扩增组织切片或细胞内微量的基因，并将其检测出来的技术。

In situ PCR combines *in situ* hybridization and PCR to detect specific genes in cells. It is a technique for amplifying and detecting trace genes in tissue sections or cells.

（三）甲基化 PCR Methylated PCR

甲基化 PCR 与常规 PCR 在原理上一致，但在引物的设计以及 DNA 样本的处理上有所不同。针对扩增的 DNA 甲基化检测区域，用重亚硫酸盐处理后，甲基化的胞嘧啶转化成尿嘧啶，非甲基化的胞嘧啶不改变。根据两个不同碱基设计两套 PCR 引物，分别针对甲基化 DNA 模板和非甲基化 DNA 模板。

Methylated PCR is consistent with conventional PCR in principle，but different in primer design and DNA sample processing. For the detection of the amplified DNA methylation region，after bisulfite treatment，methylated cytosine is converted to uracil，while non-methylated cytosine remains unchanged. Two sets of PCR primers are designed according to two different bases，for a methylated DNA template and non-methylated DNA template，respectively.

（四）实时荧光定量 PCR Real-time quantitative PCR

实时荧光定量 PCR(real-time quantitative polymerase chain reaction，RT-qPCR)是在 PCR 反应体系中加入荧光基团，利用荧光信号累积实现实时监测整个 PCR 进程，并能对起始模板进行定量分析的 PCR 技术。RT-qPCR 所使用的荧光化学物质，主要包括荧光染料（如 SYBR Green Ⅰ）和荧光探针（如 Taqman 探针）两类。RT-qPCR 不仅可以测定靶 DNA 的含量，用于临床诊断，还可以应用不同的探针检测基因突变和 SNP。

Real-time quantitative polymerase chain reaction（RT-qPCR）is a real-time quantitative PCR system in which fluorescent groups are added，the whole process of PCR can be monitored in real time by the accumulation of fluorescent signals，and the initial template can be quantitatively analyzed. RT-qPCR requires fluorescent probes. RT-qPCR can not only determine the content of target DNA for clinical diagnosis，but also detect gene mutation and afford SNP analysis with different probes.

(五) 多重引物 PCR　Multiplex PCR

多重引物 PCR(multiplex PCR)是在同一扩增体系内加入多对引物,同时扩增多个基因片段的 PCR 技术。优点是通过一次扩增可诊断几种疾病或同一疾病的几个不同的基因突变。

Multiplex primer PCR is a technique in which multiple pairs of primers are added to the same amplification system and multiple gene fragments are amplified at the same time. The advantage of this technique is that it can diagnose several diseases or several different gene mutations of the same disease using one amplification system.

(六) 套式 PCR　Nested PCR

套式 PCR 又称巢式 PCR(nested PCR),是对靶 DNA 片段设计两套引物系统,第一套引物扩增 15～30 个循环,再用扩增的 DNA 片段内设定的第二套引物扩增 15～30 个循环,可使目的 DNA 序列得到高效扩增。套式 PCR 可减少引物的非特异性扩增,减少 PCR 的误诊率。

In nested PCR，two sets of primer systems for target DNA fragments are designed. The first set of primers amplifies 15 to 30 cycles，followed by amplification for 15 to 30 cycles using the second set of primers in the amplified DNA fragments，so that the target DNA sequence can be amplified efficiently. Nested PCR can reduce the non-specific amplification of primers，increase the specific amplification，and reduce the misdiagnosis rate of PCR.

三、应用 PCR 技术检测性别决定基因

SRY 基因位于人类 Y 染色体的短臂上,编码 Y 染色体性别决定区(sex-determining region Y，SRY)蛋白。通过 PCR 反应检查 *SRY* 基因是否缺失,有助于性别鉴定和性连锁遗传病的筛查。

The sex-determining region Y protein is encoded by the *SRY* gene，which is located on the short arm of the Y chromosome. The analysis of the *SRY* gene is necessary for male sex identification and the screening of sex-linked diseases.

(一) 仪器与试剂　Required equipment and reagents

细胞裂解液、20 mg/ml 蛋白酶 K、70％乙醇、10×PCR 缓冲液、4×dNTPs、Taq DNA 聚合酶(5 U/μl)、引物 1(10 nmol/l)、引物 2(10 nmol/l)、DNA 分子量标记、上样缓冲液、离心管、PCR 管、PCR 扩增仪、电泳装置和凝胶成像系统。

Cell lysis buffer，20 mg/ml Proteinase K，70％ Ethanol，10 × PCR buffer、4 × dNTPs、Taq DNA Polymerase(5 U/μl)、primers(10 nmol/L)、DNA marker，loading buffer，centrifuge tubes，PCR tubes，PCR thermal cycler，Electrophoresis apparatus，gel imaging systems.

（二）**操作步骤　Protocols**

（1）DNA 模板制备：外周血提取 DNA　Blood DNA extraction

1）将 20 μl 20 mg/ml 蛋白酶 K 加入 0.2 ml 抗凝全血中，混匀。

Add 20 μl of 20 mg/ml proteinase K to 0.2 ml whole blood and mix with a pipette.

2）向上述混合液中加入 200 μl DNA 细胞裂解液，混匀后，70℃放置 10 min。

Add 200 μl cell lysis buffer to the blood lysate，mix，and incubate for 10 minutes at 70℃.

3）DNA 的提取（参见"真核细胞基因组 DNA 的提取"）。

DNA extraction（see "Genomic DNA extraction from eukaryotic cells"）.

（2）PCR 反应体系配制及扩增 Preparation and amplification of the PCR system

1）PCR 反应总体积 50 μl，取一 PCR 管，依次加入：

Add the following PCR reagents to one PCR tube. The total volume is 50 μl.

10×PCR buffer	5 μl
dNTPs	5 μl
Primer 1	2.5 μl
Primer 2	2.5 μl
Template DNA	10 μl
Taq DNA	2.5 U
Purified water	up to 50 μl

2）将 PCR 管放入 PCR 扩增仪上，反应条件为 94℃变性 10 min 后，94℃变性 45 s、55℃退火 45 s、72℃延伸 90 s 共 30 个循环；最末一个循环结束后，72℃再延伸 10 min。

Place the PCR tubes into a PCR thermal cycler. Follow the program：initial denaturation at 94℃ for 10 minutes; followed by 30 cycles of denaturation at 94℃ for 45 seconds，annealing at 55℃ for 45 seconds，and extension at 72℃ for 90 seconds; with a final extension at 72℃ for 10 minutes.

（3）PCR 扩增产物电泳检测 Detection of amplified products by electrophoresis

取 PCR 扩增产物 10 μl 与 2 μl 上样缓冲液混合后，与 DNA Marker 同时进行琼脂糖凝胶电泳。电泳结束后，取出凝胶置于凝胶成像系统上观察。

Mix 10 μl of the PCR amplification products with 2 μl of loading buffer and perform agarose gel electrophoresis simultaneously with a DNA Marker. After electrophoresis，observe the gel using a gel imaging system.

（三）**附录　Appendix**

引物 1 序列为 SRY1：5′- GATCAGCAAGCAGCTGGGATACCAGTG - 3′；引物 2 序列为 SRY2：5′- CTGTAGCGGTCCCGTTGCTGCGGTG - 3′。

The sequence of primer1 is：SRY1，5′- GATCAGCAAGCAGCTGGGATACCAGTG -

$3'$; the sequence of primer2 is：SRY2, $5'-$ CTGTAGCGGTCCCGTTGCTGCGGTG $- 3'$

（四）注意事项　Notes

（1）引物设计需要根据以下原则：①引物的长度保持在 $18\sim24$ bp,引物过短将影响产物的特异性,而引物过长将影响产物的合成效率；②GC 含量应保持在 $45\%\sim60\%$；③ $5'$ 和 $3'$ 端的引物间不能形成互补。

The primer design principles include keeping the length of primers between 18 and 24 bp, keeping the GC content between 45% and 60%, ensure lack of complementarity between the $5'$ and $3'$ primers.

（2）保证扩增体系成分一致性。多个样本检测时,将共用的扩增试剂预混合后分成几个反应体系,然后加入不同的模板 DNA。

The components of the amplification system should be consistent. When multiple samples are detected, the common amplification reagents are pre-mixed and divided into several reaction systems, followed by the addition of different template.

第三节 ◎ 基因芯片技术
Gene chips assay

基因芯片(gene chips)又称 DNA 芯片(DNA chips)或 DNA 微阵列(DNA microarray),以 DNA 分子杂交技术为基础,将许多已知的、特定的寡核苷酸或基因片段作为探针,有序地、高密度地排列在玻璃、硅片或尼龙膜等载体上。对待测样品 DNA 或由 RNA 通过 RT - PCR 扩增得到的 cDNA 进行荧光分子标记,并与芯片上的探针杂交,再经过激光共聚焦荧光扫描系统扫描,检测探针分子杂交信号强度,通过计算机系统对荧光信号综合分析获得样品中大量基因序列及表达的信息。通过设计不同的探针阵列、使用特定的分析方法可使该技术具有多种不同的应用价值。如基因表达谱测定、突变检测、多态性分析、基因组文库作图及杂交测序等。

Gene chips, also known as DNA chips or DNA microarray, are based on DNA molecular hybridization technology. Many known and specific oligonucleotides or gene fragments are arranged on glass, silicon, or nylon membranes in an orderly and high-density manner, as probes to prepare the DNA microarray. DNA microarray is used for fluorescence analysis of DNA samples, or a cDNA amplified by RNA through RT - PCR is hybridized with probes on the chip, followed by scanning by a confocal laser fluorescence scanning system, to detect the intensity of the hybridization signal of probes. A large number of gene sequences and expression information in samples have been obtained through comprehensive analysis of fluorescence signals using a computer system. By designing different probe arrays and using specific analytical methods, the technique can be applied in many different fields, such as gene expression profiling, mutation detection, polymorphism analysis, genomic library mapping, and hybridization sequencing.

基因芯片技术可以一次性对样品大量序列进行检测和分析,从而解决了传统核酸杂交技术操作繁杂、自动化程度低、操作序列数量少、检测效率低等不足。将大量(通常每平方厘米点阵密度高于400)探针分子固定于支持物上后与标记的样品分子进行杂交,通过检测每个探针分子的杂交信号强度进而获取样品分子的数量和序列信息(图7-2)。

Gene chips can detect and analyze a large number of samples at one time, thus overcoming the shortcomings of traditional nucleic acid imprinting hybridization technologies (Southern hybridization and Northern hybridization), such as complicated operation, low automation, small number of operation sequences, low detection efficiency. A large number of probe molecules (usually more than 400 dot density per square centimeter) are fixed on the support and hybridized with the labeled sample molecules (Fig. 7-2).

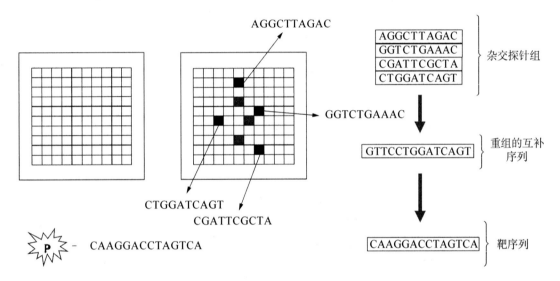

图7-2 基因芯片技术的原理
Fig. 7-2 Principle of gene chips

一、基因芯片使用的基本流程 Gene chips procedure

基因芯片技术的主要步骤包括芯片制备、样品制备、杂交反应及信号检测和结果分析。

The gene chips include four main steps: chip preparation, sample preparation, hybridization reaction, signal detection and analysis.

(一)待测样本的制备 Sample preparation

基因芯片的样本来自于两个方面:其一是直接从组织和细胞中分离纯化DNA,并对待测样本中的DNA进行特异扩增;其二是提纯RNA,并进行反转录以及cDNA扩增。在DNA扩增的过程中需要完成样本的标记。目前,样品标记常采用荧光标记法,也可用生物素或放射性同位素。

DNA samples isolated from tissue and cells are specifically amplified or cDNAs are reverse transcribed from RNA by RT-PCR. In the process of DNA amplification, the labeling of samples needs to be completed.

(二) 杂交反应　Hybridization reaction

基因芯片的分子杂交与 Southern 杂交的方法一致。由于芯片的表面会干扰靶分子与探针的结合,因此需要相应地延长杂交时间或增加靶分子浓度。

Hybridization of gene chips is consistent with Southern hybridization. It is necessary to prolong the hybridization time or increase the concentration of the target molecule to overcome the interference of the chip's surface.

(三) 检测分析　Detection and analysis

基因芯片分子杂交信号的检测和分析通过阅读仪及其分析软件来完成。阅读仪可分为激光共聚焦扫描和电荷耦合器件(charge-coupled device,CCD)两种。前者分辨率和灵敏度较高,可获取高质量的图像和数据,但扫描速度较慢,而且价格昂贵。后者的特点与之相反。目前常用的是激光共聚焦扫描仪。

基因芯片杂交实验产生庞大的杂交信息,需要生物信息学手段的支持。借助读取和分析杂交信号的应用软件以及与网络公共数据库连接进行数据分析的应用软件,可以高效获得研究对象的有效信息。

Confocal laser scanning molecular hybridization signal acquisition and a bioinformatics analytical software are used to analyze the huge amount of hybridization information.

二、基因表达谱芯片技术　Gene expression profiling by DNA microarray technology

基因表达谱芯片技术提供了一种高通量的方法,可以同时分析成千上万个基因的表达。基因表达谱芯片技术采用 cDNA 或寡核苷酸片段作探针,固化在芯片上。将待测样品(处理组)与对照样品的 mRNA 以两种不同的荧光分子进行标记,然后同时与芯片进行杂交。基因芯片每个点可以获得不同波长下的荧光强度值及其比值,并得到直观的显色图。通过分析两种样品与探针杂交的荧光强度的比值,来检测基因表达水平的变化,以研究不同样本间基因表达差异。目前常用的荧光染料是 Cy3(绿色)和 Cy5(红色)(图 7 - 3)。

Gene expression profiling by DNA microarray technology provides a high-throughput approach to analyze the expression of tens of thousands of genes simultaneously. The cDNA or oligonucleotide fragments are used as probes and immobilized on the chip. The mRNAs of the samples of the treatment group and the control group are labeled with two different fluorescent molecules and hybridized with the chip. The fluorescence intensity and ratio values at different wavelengths can be obtained at each point of the gene chip and a visual chromogram is generated. By analyzing the ratio of the fluorescence intensity of the hybridization between two samples and the probe, the changes in gene expression level are detected and used to study the difference in gene expression between different samples. Cy3 (green) and Cy5 (red) are fluorescent dyes that are commonly used (Fig. 7 - 3).

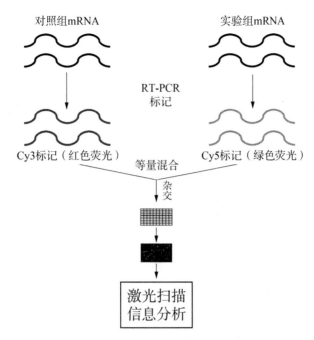

图 7-3 基因表达谱芯片技术

Fig. 7-3 Gene Expression Profiling by DNA Microarray Technology

三、SNP 芯片 SNP chips

单核苷酸多态性(single nucleotide polymorphism，SNP)是最简单、最常见、分布最为广泛，也是多态性最为丰富的遗传多态类型之一，可以通过测序技术、质谱分析等技术进行分析，以求找到疾病相对应的 SNP 位点或者是进行个性化药物治疗研究。2007 年，包括全基因组 SNP 位点探针的 SNP 芯片开始用于全基因组 SNP 分析，通过基因分型信息可以鉴别杂合性缺失(loss of heterozygosity，lOH)、单亲二倍体病(uniparental disomy，UPD)及嵌合现象等。SNP 芯片检测通量很大，一次可以检测几十万到几百万个 SNP 位点，精准性可以达到 99.9%以上，而且检测费用相对较低。

Single-nucleotide polymorphism analysis is a hotspots in gene mutation research. SNPs can be analyzed by sequencing, mass spectrometry, and other techniques to identify the corresponding mutation sites in diseases or to conduct personalized drug treatment research. Whole-genome SNP chips contain the whole-genome SNP locus probes for SNP analysis. Loss of heterozygosity (LOH), uniparental diploid disease (UPD), and chimerism (20% chimerism can be accurately detected) can be identified based on genotyping information. SNP chips have a large detection flux, which can detect hundreds of thousands to millions of SNP loci at a time; moreover, the accuracy of this technology can reach more than 99.9% and its cost is relatively low.

四、MicroRNA 芯片　MicroRNA chips

MicroRNA(miRNA)是真核生物体内一类具有基因表达调控功能的非编码小分子RNA。miRNAs通过对基因的调控,在生物发育、细胞增殖和凋亡及肿瘤发生过程中发挥重要作用。标记不同样本中的总 RNA,然后与 miRNA 芯片杂交,通过扫描芯片上信号的强度,计算出样品中 miRNAs 的表达量,从而了解样品间差异表达的 miRNAs。

MicroRNAs are non-coding small RNAs with gene expression regulation function in eukaryotic organisms. MicroRNAs play an important role in biological development, cell proliferation, apoptosis, and tumorigenesis through gene regulation. Total RNA samples from different samples are marked and then hybridized with the microRNA chip. The expression of microRNAs in the samples is calculated by scanning the intensity of the signal on the chip, to determine which microRNAs are abnormal in the samples.

五、基因芯片的应用　Applications of gene chips

（一）基因表达分析　Gene expression analysis
基因芯片技术是基因筛选的有效方法,揭示基因突变诱导人类疾病的病因以及发生机制。

Gene chips assay can be used for gene screening to examine the etiology and pathogenesis of human diseases induced by gene mutation.

（二）基因突变检测　Detection of gene mutation
基因芯片是高效检测基因突变的方法。经典的研究多采用 PCR - SSCP、手工或自动测序、异源双链分析、蛋白截短检测等方法,缺点为限制了在大规模研究中的应用。基因芯片克服了经典研究方法步骤繁琐、工作量大、工作效率较低等不足。

The gene chips assay can overcome the shortcomings of the classical methods for studying gene mutation, such as cumbersome steps, heavy workload, and low efficiency.

（三）药物筛选　Drug screening
应用基因芯片技术不仅能够分析用药前后机体不同组织、器官基因表达的差异,而且可以筛选与药物结合的药物蛋白或核酸。基因芯片技术大大提高药物筛选、靶基因鉴别和新药测试的速度,降低了研究成本。

The gene chips assay can be used not only to analyze the differences in gene expression in different tissues and organs before and after medication, but also to screen drug-binding proteins or nucleic acids. The gene chips assay greatly improves the speed of drug screening, target gene identification, and new drug testing, and reduces the cost of research.

（四）在其他领域中的应用　Other fields
随着人类基因组计划的完成,人类医学将从群体医学向个体医学过度。利用基因芯片高通量的测试手段可以确定与药物代谢相关的基因多态性,进而辅助临床用药。

High-throughput microarray testing can be used to identify gene polymorphisms associated with drug metabolism，which is helpful for personalized therapy. Gene chips can also diagnose different pathogens of the same disease，and can be used for clinical guidance.

第四节 ◎ 基因测序技术
Gene sequencing technology

遗传病的本质是由于基因突变及其表观突变、染色体畸变导致的。基因水平的大部分改变可以通过测序来检测。从 19 世纪 70 年代发明的 Sanger 测序到近几年的单分子测序技术对基因组研究，疾病医疗研究，药物研发等领域起到了巨大的推动作用。已经成为遗传病临床分子诊断的重要技术手段。基因测序技术经历了三代的发展历程，目前三代技术都在应用。

The essence of genetic disease is gene mutation，epigenetic mutation，and chromosomal aberration. Most changes at the gene level can be detected by sequencing. From the Sanger sequencing invented in the 1970s to the single-molecule sequencing technology of recent years，this technology has played a tremendous role in the fields of genome research，disease-related medical research，and pharmaceutical development. It has become an important technique for the clinical molecular diagnosis of genetic diseases. The gene sequencing technology has gone through three generations of development. At present，three generations of technology are being applied.

一、第一代 Sanger 测序 First-generation Sanger sequencing

主要基于双脱氧终止法的测序原理。利用一种 DNA 聚合酶来延伸结合在待定序列模板上的引物，直到掺入一种链终止核苷酸为止。每次测序反应由一套 4 个单独的 PCR 反应构成，每个反应含有所有 4 种脱氧核苷酸三磷酸（dNTP），并混入限量的某一种不同的双脱氧核苷三磷酸（ddNTP）。ddNTP 使延长的寡聚核苷酸选择性地在 G、A、T 或 C 处终止，终止点处的 ddNTP 即为模板链的核苷酸。每个 PCR 反应得到一组长短不一的链终止产物。通过高分辨率变性凝胶电泳分离大小不同的片段，凝胶处理后可用 X 线胶片放射自显影或非同位素标记进行检测。人类基因组计划就是基于一代测序技术。第一代的 Sanger 测序技术的优点是测序读长长，能达到 800～1 000 bp；只需要几十分钟即可完成一次测序，测序准确度高准确性高达 99.999%，目前仍是测序的"金标准"；缺点是通量低、成本高，影响了其真正大规模的应用。

Sanger sequencing is mainly based on the sequencing principle of the termination of deoxygenation. A DNA polymerase is used to extend the primers bound to the template of the undetermined sequence until a strand termination nucleotide is incorporated. Each sequencing reaction consists of a set of four separate PCR reactions，each containing all four kinds of deoxynucleotide triphosphate（dNTP）mixed with a limited amount of a different kind of dideoxynucleotide triphosphate（ddNTP）. The ddNTP selectively terminates the extended oligonucleotides at G，A，T，or C，and the ddNTP at the termination point is the nucleotide of the template chain. Each PCR reaction yields a set of chain-termination products of different lengths. High-resolution denaturing gel electrophoresis is then used to separate fragments of different sizes. After gel treatment，X-ray optical films are used for autoradiography or non-isotope labeling. This sequencing technology has the characteristics of high accuracy and rapidity. Sanger sequencing with 99.999% accuracy is the "gold standard" for sequencing.

二、第二代高通量测序　Second-generation high-throughput sequencing

第二代高通量测序又称为下一代测序（next generation sequencing，NGS），其基本原理是边合成边测序。用不同颜色的荧光标记 4 种不同的 dNTP，当 DNA 聚合时，通过捕捉新合成的末端标记来确定 DNA 的序列。现有的技术平台主要包括 Roche/454 FLX、Illumina/Solexa Genome Analyzer 和 Applied Biosystems SOLID system。具体流程如下：酶切 DNA 成小片段加接头，固定于介质上，扩增待测片段，加入带有荧光标记的 dNTP 合成待测片段互补链，收集逐步合成的荧光信号，生物信息学组装信号。二代测序可以实现全基因组 DNA 的测序，也可以针对全基因组外显子区域 DNA 捕捉、富集后进行高通量测序。比较成熟的二代测序技术有两个共同的特点：①需要把基因组 DNA 切割成比较短的片段（200～500 bp）；②把这些 DNA 片段固定在支撑物上，让不同片段处于相对独立的空间位置。这两个特点可以让大量的 DNA 短片段同时被测序，大大提高了测序的效率。

Second-generation high-throughput sequencing also known as next-generation sequencing(NGS). The basic principle of the second-generation sequencing technology is to perform sequencing while synthesizing. Four different dNTPs are labeled with different colors of fluorescence. After DNA polymerization，the DNA sequence is determined by capturing newly synthesized end labels. The existing platforms for this technology include mainly the Roche/454 FLX，Illumina/Solexa Genome Analyzer，and Applied Biosystems SOLID systems. The specific process is as follows：enzymatic digestion of DNA into small fragments and joints，fixation on the medium，amplification of the fragments to be measured，addition of dNTPs with fluorescent labels to synthesize complementary chains of the fragments to be measured，collection of gradually synthesized fluorescent signals，and assembly of bioinformatics signals. Second-generation sequencing can realize whole-genome DNA sequencing，as well as high-throughput sequencing for DNA capture and enrichment in exonic regions of the whole genome. The two general features of the well-established NGS methods are：① the fragmentation of genomic DNA（200 to 500 bp）and ② the subsequent immobilization of spatially separated template DNA fragments on a solid surface prior to sequencing.

三、第三代单分子测序　Third-generation single-molecule sequencing

单分子 DNA 测序时，不需要经过 PCR 扩增就可以实现对每一条 DNA 分子的单独测序。第三代测序技术已经应用在基因组测序、甲基化研究、突变鉴定（包括 SNP）等 3 个方面。

三代测序目前共有两种方法。一种方法是单分子荧光测序，以单分子光谱技术（single-molecule spectroscopy，SMS）和单分子实时（single-molecule real-time，SMRT）测序技术为代表。DNA 聚合酶固定在几十纳米的纳米孔处，带有不同荧光标记的脱氧核苷酸渗入 DNA 链时荧光加强，形成化学键后荧光消失，同时 A、T、C、G 聚合的速度也是不一样的。因此，显微镜可以实时记录荧光的强度及停滞时间的变化，实现单分子 DNA 测序。另一种方法是纳米孔测序，根据单个核酸聚合物通过直径非常细小的纳米孔时，每种碱基的带电性质不一样，通过电信号的差异就能检测出通过的碱基类别，从而实现测序。

In single-molecule sequencing, the individual sequencing of each DNA molecule can be achieved without the PCR amplification. The third-generation sequencing technology has been applied in genome sequencing, methylation research, and mutation identification (SNP detection).

The third-generation sequencing currently employ two methods. One method is single-molecule fluorescence sequencing, which is represented by single-molecule spectroscopy (SMS) and single-molecule real-time (SMRT) sequencing. DNA polymerase is immobilized in the nanopore of tens of nanometers. Fluorescence is enhanced by the penetration of deoxynucleotides with different fluorescence labels into DNA strands, and fluorescence disappears after the formation of chemical bonds. At the same time, the speed of A, T, C, and G polymerization is also different. Therefore, microscopy can be used to record the changes in fluorescence intensity and stagnation time in real time and realize single-molecule DNA sequencing. Another method is nanopore sequencing method, which based on the placement of a single nucleic acid polymer into a pore with a very small diameter. Each base has different charged properties, and the difference in electrical signals can be detected through the base type, thus achieving sequencing.

（吴　丹）

第八章 染色体分析相关的实验
Chromosome-analysis-related experiments

染色体是细胞与分子联系的重要桥梁，染色体的研究在遗传学和医学研究中被广泛重视及应用。尤其是染色体畸变有关的各类遗传病的研究使临床分析上了一个新的台阶。

在染色体分析技术中，染色体非显带技术相对较简单，通常采用外周血中的淋巴细胞。产前诊断时，胎儿可采用羊膜液中的羊膜细胞或胎盘绒毛膜细胞。染色体显带技术是在非显带染色体的基础上发展起来的，能显示染色体本身更细微的结构，有助于精准识别每一条染色体及诊断染色体异常疾病。随着分子细胞遗传学技术的发展，可利用DNA探针来定位染色体上特定的基因和DNA序列，如荧光原位杂交技术，可以鉴别经典细胞遗传学方法所难以识别的微小标记染色体、微小缺失和复杂易位等。

As chromosomes are important bridges between cells and molecules，the study of chromosomes has been widely regarded and used in genetics and medical research.

In chromosome-analysis techniques，peripheral blood chromosome preparation is currently the most widely used cytogenetic diagnostic technique. The chromosome banding technique can pinpoint the finer structure of the chromosome itself，which helps to identify each chromosome accurately and diagnose diseases caused by chromosomal abnormalities. Via the application of molecular cytogenetics techniques，cloned DNA probes can also be used to locate specific genes and DNA sequences on chromosomes.

第一节 ◎ 人类染色体标本的制备
Human chromosome preparation

一、概述 Overview

在一般的生理状态下，全血中含有红细胞和白细胞。红细胞没有核，无分裂能力；白细胞虽有细胞核存在，但是在外周血中处于静止期（G_0），因此要使白细胞从间期进入分裂期必须加刺激药物。

目前最常用的促使分裂的药品是植物血凝素（phytohemagglutinin，PHA），它能使白细胞中的淋巴细胞和单核细胞转化为具有分裂作用的母细胞，这就为染色体的制备创造了条件。在PHA的作用下，处在G_0期的淋巴细胞可转化成淋巴母细胞，重新进入增殖周期进行有丝分裂。当体外培养至70 h左右时,大多数淋巴细胞处于第二增殖周期内,此时用秋水仙素(colchicine)处理细胞可使正在分裂的细胞都停止在中期,再经低渗处理、固定、染色,获取中期分裂相细胞的染色体标本,可在显微镜下拍照进行核型分析,或用计算机进行图像分析。

In the general physiological state, the whole blood contains red and white blood cells, which are all undivided interphase cells. Erythrocytes have no nucleus and no ability to divide. Although leukocytes have a nucleus, they are already in the resting phase (G_0) in the peripheral blood. Therefore, it is necessary to add a stimulating drug to drive leukocytes out of interphase, to enter the dividing phase.

The most commonly used drug that causes division is phytohemagglutinin (PHA), which converts lymphocytes and monocytes in leukocytes into metrocytes with dividing effects, thus creating the conditions that are necessary for chromosome preparation. Under the action of PHA, the lymphocytes in the G_0 phase can be transformed into lymphoblasts and re-enter the proliferation cycle for mitosis. When cultured *in vitro* for about 70 hours, most lymphocytes are in the second proliferation cycle. Treatment of cells with colchicine allows cells that are dividing to arrest division in metaphase, followed by hypotonic treatment, fixation, and staining, to obtain metaphase meristematic cells. Chromosome specimens can be photographed under a microscope for karyotyping or image analysis using a computer.

二、人类染色体标本的制备 Human chromosome preparation

(一)仪器与试剂 Required equipment and reagents

离心机、离心管、冰玻片、恒温水浴箱、恒温培养箱、光学显微镜、RPMI 1640、胎牛血清、肝素(500 U/ml)、秋水仙素(5 μg/ml)、植物血凝素(PHA)、固定液(甲醇:冰乙酸为3:1)、0.075 mol/L KCl溶液、Giemsa染液、pH 6.8 PBS、5%NaHCO₃。

Centrifuge, centrifuge tubes, slides, constant-temperature water bath, constant-temperature incubator, optical microscope, RPMI 1640, FBS, 500 U/ml heparin, 5 μg/ml colchicine, phytohemagglutinin (PHA), fixative (ratio of methanol to glacial acetic acid, 3:1), hypotonic 0.075 mol/L KCl, Giemsa staining solution, PBS (pH 6.8), 5% NaHCO₃.

(二)操作步骤 Protocols

(1) 将0.5 ml外周血加入10 ml含有PHA和10%胎牛血清的RPMI 1640培养基中,37℃、5% CO₂的培养箱中培养72 h。

Incubate approximately 0.5 ml of heparinized whole blood in a centrifuge tube with 10 ml RPMI 1640 (PHA, 10% FBS) at 37℃ and 5% CO₂ for 72 hours.

(2) 在终止培养前4 h,加入秋水仙素(终浓度为0.07 μg/ml),轻轻摇匀。放回培养箱内,继续培养4 h。

Add colchicine to the centrifuge tube (the final concentration of colchicine is 0.07 μg/ml) and gently shake. Incubate the culture for an additional 4 hours.

（3）收获细胞：用吸管充分吹打瓶壁，吸取培养物移入离心管内，1 000 r/min 离心 10 min，弃上清液。

Transfer the culture to a centrifuge tube and centrifuge at 1 000 r/min for 10 minutes, and discard the supernatant.

（4）低渗处理：加 8 ml 预温（37℃）的 0.075 mol/L KCl 低渗液，用吸管打匀使细胞悬浮于低渗液中，放在 37℃ 恒温水浴锅中，静置 15～20 min，使白细胞膨胀，染色体分散（精准的低渗时间应自行摸索）。

Resuspend the cells with 8 ml of pre-warmed hypotonic 0. 075 mol/L KCl, mix, and incubate at 37℃ for 15 to 20 minutes. The hypotonic solution causes the cell to swell and the chromosomes to seperate (the exact hypotonic time should depend on pre-experiment).

（5）预固定：低渗处理完成后，加入现配制固定液 1 ml，吹打均匀。1 000 r/min 离心 10 min。

Add 1 ml of the fresh fixative made up of 1 part acetic acid and 3 parts methanol, mix, and centrifuge at 1 000 r/min for 10 minutes.

（6）固定：弃上清液，并一滴滴加入新配的固定液 8 ml，吹打均匀，1 000 r/min 离心 10 min。

Remove the supernatant, add 8 ml of fresh fixative drop-by-drop, and mix well. Centrifuge at 1 000 r/min for 10 minutes.

（7）再固定：再加入新配固定液 8 ml，吹打均匀，静置 30 min，1 000 r/min 离心 8～10 min。

Remove the supernatant, add 8 ml of fresh fixative drop-by-drop, and mix well. Incubate at room temperature for 30 minutes, centrifuge at 1 000 r/min for 8 to 10 minutes, and discard the supernatant.

（8）制片：视细胞多少，加入适量（0.5～1.0 ml）新配固定液制成细胞悬液，将细胞悬液 2～3 滴，滴到清洁的冰玻片上，在乙醇灯火焰上来回过几下（勿全烤干），空气中晾干。

Resuspend the cell pellet in a small volume (0. 5 to 1. 0 ml) of fresh fixative, to prepare a cell suspension. Drop 2 to 3 drops of the cell suspension onto a clean slide and allow to dry in the air after a few passes over the flame of an ethanol lamp.

（9）染色：晾干的标本用 Giemsa 染液染色 8～10 min，自来水冲洗，晾干。

Stain the slide with Giemsa staining solution for 8 to 10 minutes, wash with water, and allow to air dry.

（10）镜检：将制备好的染色体玻片放置到显微镜下，先用低倍镜找到分散良好的分裂相，然后换高倍镜、油镜，认真观察。

Place the slides under a microscope, find well-dispersed chromosomes using a low-magnification lens (20×), and observe with a high-magnification lens (40×); finally, observe with a 100× oil-immersion objective.

（三）注意事项 Notes

（1）秋水仙素浓度与处理时间需最佳。如果浓度太低,处理时间太短,则分裂象少;浓度太高,处理时间太长,则分裂象虽多,但因染色体缩得太短而形态特征模糊。

Improper selection of colchicine concentration and treatment time can lead to an abnormal chromosome morphology.

（2）培养温度应严格控制在(37.0±0.5)℃。

The culture temperature should be strictly controlled at (37.0±0.5)℃.

（3）低渗一步极为重要,关系到染色体分散的好坏,因此低渗液的浓度与低渗的时间应掌握好。

It is necessary to control the concentration and time of the hypotonic solution.

（4）离心速度不宜过高,速度太高细胞团不易打散,反之分裂相易丢失。

The speed of the centrifuge should not be too high or too low.

（5）固定液应临用时新鲜配制,固定时一定要彻底吹匀,若吹打不够则细胞在玻片上成堆;反之则细胞易碎,以至染色体数目不完整。

The fixative should be prepared freshly at the time of use and must be mixed very well.

第二节 ◉ 染色体 G 显带技术
G banding

染色体显带技术(chromosome banding)是在非显带染色体的基础上发展起来的,能显示染色体本身更细微的结构。自 20 世纪 60 年代末以来,染色体显带技术得到了很大的发展。这一技术的应用,可以精准识别 23 对不同类型的染色体,并能识别同一号染色体上的不同区带。从而提高了染色体核型分析的精准度,为临床上某些疾病的诊断提供了更有效的手段。

显带染色体是染色体标本经过一定程序处理,并用特定染料染色,使染色体沿其长轴显现明暗或深浅相间的带纹,称为染色体带;这种使染色体显带的技术,称为显带技术。通过显带技术,使各号染色体都显现出独特的带纹,这就构成了染色体的带型。每对同源染色体的带型基本相同而且稳定,不同对染色体的带型不同。20 世纪 70 年代以来,显带技术得到了很大发展,在众多的显带(Q 带、G 带、C 带、R 带、T 带)技术中,G 带是目前应用最广泛的一种。因为它主要是被 Giemsa 染料染色后而显带,故称之为 G 显带技术(Giemsa banding, G banding)。一套单倍体染色体带纹数有 320 条带。70 年代后期,由于技术的改进,可以从早期、前中期、晚前期细胞得到更长、带纹更丰富的染色体。一套单倍体染色体即可显示 550～850 条或更多的带纹,称为高分辨显带染色体(high resolution banding chromosome, HRBC)。

The chromosomal banding technique was developed based on non-banding chromosomes and can accurately identify 23 pairs of different types of chromosomes and recognize different regions on the same chromosome. The G banding is currently the most widely used. This method improves the accuracy of karyotype analyses and is widely used in the diagnosis and research of chromosomal diseases.

一、概述　Overview

关于 G 带的形成机制,迄今尚不十分清楚。有人认为,在胰蛋白酶的作用下,蛋白质不均匀丢失是 G 带产生的原因。染色体上的蛋白质经处理而丢失后的区域呈现出浅染(浅带)。而染色体上蛋白质和 DNA 结合牢固的区域,由于蛋白质丢失少而呈现深染(深带)。还有人认为,染色体经胰蛋白酶消化后,染色体的核蛋白破坏,这些区域裸露的 DNA 分子的磷酸基团能与 Giemsa 染料中的天青和甲基蓝等噻嗪分子结合而使染色体着色。也有人认为,染色体上 T-A 和 C-G 碱基对的含量和分布不同,与染色体上深浅带的形成有关。T-A 碱基对较多的区域,易与 Giemsa 染料结合而染成深色区带;而 C-G 碱基对较多的区域则相反,染成浅染区带。总之,目前说法较多,主要概括为三种观点,即显带是由于:①DNA 的作用;②蛋白质的作用;③DNA、染料和蛋白质三者之间相互作用的结果,都有待于进一步研究。人染色体标本经胰蛋白酶、NaOH、柠檬酸盐或尿素等试剂处理后,再用 Giemsa 染色,可使每条染色体上显示出深浅交替的横纹,这就是染色体的 G 显带技术。

G 显带制备方法简便易行,标本可长期保存,带纹清晰,成本低廉,制备周期短,普通光学显微镜即可观察。故已成为研究分析染色体的常规方法之一。

Human chromosome specimens are treated with reagents such as trypsin, NaOH, citrate, or urea, and then stained with Giemsa. Each chromosome displays alternating horizontal stripes, which are the G bands of the chromosome. The formation mechanism of the G band is not fully understood, but can be summarized as three main viewpoints: the banding is caused by the role of DNA, the role of proteins, and the results of interaction between DNA, dyes, and proteins. These are all to be further studied and discussed.

二、G 显带　G banding

(一) 仪器与试剂　Required equipment and reagents

2.5% 胰蛋白酶原液、0.25% 胰蛋白酶工作液、生理盐水、Giemsa 原液、Giemsa 工作液、1 mol/L PBS(pH 4.0~4.5)、普通光学显微镜、37℃恒温水浴箱、染色缸。

Trypsin stock solution (2.5%), 0.25% trypsin working solution, normal saline, Giemsa stock solution, Giemsa working solution, 1 mol/L PBS (pH 4.0 to 4.5), optical microscope, 37℃ constant-temperature water bath, coplin jars.

(二) 操作步骤　Protocols

(1) 将常规制备的人染色体玻片标本(未染色的白片)置于 70℃烤箱中处理 2 h,然后转入 37℃培养箱中备用,一般在第 3~7 天进行显带。

Place the chromosome slides (without staining) in an oven at 70℃ for 2 hours, and transfer to a 37℃ incubator for 3 to 7 days.

(2) 取 0.25% 胰蛋白酶溶液 5 ml,倒入染色缸中,加入 45 ml 生理盐水,用 1 mol/L HCl 和 1 mol/L NaOH 及酚红调节胰蛋白酶溶液至 pH 7.0~7.4。

Add 5 ml of 0.25% trypsin solution and 45 ml of normal saline to the same staining Coplin. Adjust the trypsin solution to a pH in the range of 7.0 to 7.4 with 1 mol/L HCl, 1 mol/L NaOH, and phenol red.

（3）将配好的胰蛋白酶工作液放入37℃恒温水浴箱中预温。

Pre-warm the prepared trypsin working solution in a 37℃ constant-temperature water bath.

（4）将玻片标本浸入胰蛋白酶液中，不断摆动使胰蛋白酶的作用均匀，处理1～2 min（精确的时间需自行摸索）。

Immerse the slides in trypsin solution for 1 to 2 minutes and oscillate continuously, to render the action of trypsin uniform.

（5）立即取出玻片，放入生理盐水中漂洗2次。

Immediately take the slides out and rinse twice in normal saline.

（6）将玻片浸入37℃预温的Giemsa工作液中染色10 min左右。

Immerse the slides in a 37℃ pre-warmed Giemsa working solution for about 10 minutes.

（7）自来水冲洗（用细水小心冲洗），空气晾干。

Wash carefully with water and air dry.

（8）镜检显带效果：在低倍镜下选择分散良好、长度适中的分裂象，转换油镜观察，若染色体未出现带纹，则为显带不足；若染色体边缘发毛为显带过久，此时应根据具体情况增减胰蛋白酶处理时间重新处理一张标本。

Select well-dispersed chromosomes with good length under low magnification and under an oil-immersion objective. If there is no band on the chromosome, the trypsin treatment is insufficient. While the fuzzy chromosome is overexposed, the specimen should be reprocessed according to the specific conditions of the trypsin treatment.

（三）G 显带核型分析　G-banding karyotype analysis

传统的G显带核型分析，需将G显带中期分裂相照片上各条染色体逐一剪下，根据其大小、带型特点和着丝粒位置，依次分组、配对和排列组合，待检查无误后，贴在报告纸上，写出核型的简式（繁式）。目前，也可以通过核型分析软件辅助分析。

Prepare a photograph of the metaphase chromosomes of the Gbanding and cut each chromosome out one by one. The chromosomes are then grouped, paired, and arranged in sequence depending on their size, characteristic banding pattern, and centromere position. After being checked, paste it onto the report paper and write the karyotype. At present, karyotype analysis software can facilitate the data collection.

（四）注意事项　Notes

（1）良好的培养效果为：标本片上中期分裂象要多，且染色体分散要好。

A good culture outcome includes many metaphase cells on the slide and a good chromosomes separation.

（2）胰蛋白酶溶液需在使用前新鲜配制。

The trypsin solution needs to be prepare freshly before use.

（3）染色体长度应能适应显带分析技术的要求。

The length of the chromosome should be able to adapt to the requirements of the banding analysis technique.

（4）G显带成败之关键取决于胰蛋白酶液的浓度和处理时间之搭配，故每次进行染色体G显带时，最好先试做一张制片，摸索胰蛋白酶处理时间，以保证获得最好的染色体G显带标本。

Excellent G -banding patterns depend on the concentration of the trypsin solution and the processing time.

第三节 ◎ 姐妹染色单体交换技术
Sister chromatid exchange assay

姐妹染色单体交换（sister chromatial exchange，SCE)是染色体同源座位上复制产物间的相互交换，是同一染色体的两条单体之间发生的一类特殊的同源重组，主要在DNA合成期形成，可能与DNA双链的断裂与复制有关，SCE的发生频率可反映细胞在S期的受损程度。如果一个个体的SCE率明显增高，可表明染色体受到环境中的一定因素的影响，或是受到遗传缺陷的内在制约因素所致。

Sister chromatid exchange （SCE) is a type of special homologous recombination between two monomers on the same chromosome. The formation of SCE may be related to the cleavage and replication of DNA duplexes，and the frequency of SCE occurrence may reflect the degree of damage of cells in the S phase.

一、概述 Overview

5-溴脱氧尿嘧啶核苷(BrdU)是脱氧胸腺嘧啶核苷的类似物，在DNA链的复制过程中，可替代胸腺嘧啶。在细胞培养过程中加入BrdU，在DNA复制过程中，BrdU就能取代胸腺嘧啶而被掺入到新合成的DNA中。经过两个分裂周期后，两条姐妹染色单体中的一条由双股都含有BrdU的DNA链构成，而另一条为单股含有BrdU的DNA链。在结构上双股含BrdU的DNA螺旋化程度较低，故对染色剂亲合力低，用Giemsa染色时其单体着色浅；而只有单股含BrdU的DNA链组成的单体着色深，两条姐妹染色单体形成差别着色。当姐妹染色体间存在同源片段交换时，可根据每条单体夹杂着深浅不一的着色片段加以区分，这就是姐妹染色单体交换技术(sister chromatid exchange assay)。由于姐妹染色单体的DNA序列相同，SCE并不改变遗传物质组成，但SCE是由于染色体发生断裂和重接而产生的，因此，SCE技术通常用来检测染色体断裂频率，用来研究药物和环境因素的致畸效应。

The exchange of homologous fragments occurs at the same site between two monomers from one chromosome. When the cells are in the second division cycle，one sister chromatid consists of a DNA strand containing both 5-bromodeoxyuridine （BrdU） and the other sister chromatid is a single strand of BrdU-containing DNA. The structure of the double-stranded

BrdU-containing DNA is less helical; thus, the monomer is lightly colored when dyed with Giemsa, and only the single-stranded BrdU-containing DNA strand is darkly colored. A homologous fragment exchange between the sister chromosomes can be distinguished according to the coloring fragments of each monomer mixed with different shades. The sister chromatid exchange assay is commonly used to detect chromosome break frequency and to study the teratogenic effects of drugs and environmental factors.

二、仪器与试剂　Required equipment and reagents

RPMI 1640、PHA、肝素、2×SSC、500 μg/ml BrdU、PBS(pH 6.8)、Giemsa 染液、光学显微镜、离心机、玻片染色缸。

RPMI 1640, PHA, heparin, 2×SSC, 500 μg/ml BrdU, PBS (pH 6.8), Giemsa staining solution, microscope, centrifuge, coplin jars.

三、操作步骤　Protocols

(一)细胞培养(人外周血淋巴细胞培养)　Cell culture (human peripheral blood lymphocyte culture)

(1) 接种:无菌抽取外周血 0.2~0.3 ml(肝素抗凝),接种在 5 ml 含有 PHA 的 RPMI 1640 培养液中,37℃培养箱培养。

Peripheral whole blood (0.2 to 0.3 ml) is aseptically inoculated into 5 ml of RPMI 1640 medium containing PHA and cultured in a 37℃ incubator.

(2) 加 BrdU:培养 24 h 后加 500 μg/ml BrdU 液 0.1 ml,终浓度为 10 μg/ml,混匀后,避光培养。

After 24 hours of culture, add 0.1 ml of 500 μg/ml BrdU solution to a final concentration of 10 μg/ml. After mixing, incubate the cells in the dark.

(3) 加秋水仙素:在收获细胞前 2 h 加秋水仙素(终浓度为 0.2 μg/ml)。

Add colchicine 2 hours before the harvesting of cells. The final concentration of colchicine is 0.2 μg/ml.

(二)收获细胞和制备染色体玻片　Harvesting of cells and preparation of chromosome slides

参见"人类染色体标本的制备"。

See "human chromosome preparation".

(三)标本老化　Specimen aging

将制好的染色体玻片置 37℃培养箱 2 d 或在 60℃烤箱烤片 2 h。

Place the prepared chromosome slides in a 37℃ incubator for 2 days or in a dry oven at 60℃ for 2 hours.

(四)差别染色(紫外线照射法)　Differential dyeing (ultraviolet irradiation)

(1) 将染色体玻片置于 56℃水浴锅盖上,铺上 2×SSC 液,距 20 W 紫外灯管 6 cm 处紫外照射 30 min。

Put the chromosome slides on the top of water bath (56℃), add 2×SSC solution on the slide，and irradiate with 20 W ultraviolet for 30 minutes. The distance between the UV lamp and the slides should be about 6 cm.

（2）弃去 2×SSC 液，立即用 4℃左右的流水冲洗。

Discard the 2×SSC solution and wash immediately with water（4℃）.

（3）Giemsa 液染色 5 min(不要着色过深)，流水冲洗，干燥后镜检。

Stain with Giemsa staining solution for 5 min，wash with water，and observe under the microscope.

（五）实验结果及分析　Results and analysis

（1）选择在加入 BrdU 之后经过两个复制周期，姐妹染色单体分化着色清晰，染色体分散良好，长短合适且染色数目完整的中期分裂相，进行观察分析。

The results were analyzed via the chromosomes of two replication cycles after the addition of BrdU. The sister chromatid differentiation is clear and well-distributed，the length is appropriate，and the number is complete.

（2）SCE 交换次数判定：染色体某臂端部交换算 1 次交换，臂间交换算 2 次；着丝粒处发生交换(需排除染色体在此发生扭曲)计 1 次。

Method used for judging the number of exchanges of SCE：the exchange of one end of the chromosome is counted as one exchange and the exchange between the arms is counted twice. The exchange is performed once at the centromere，and it is necessary to exclude the distortion of the chromosome here.

（3）每个标本分析 30～50 个中期分裂相。

Analyze each specimen for 30 to 50 metaphase divisions.

（4）SCE 率计算。

SCE 率＝累计互换数／观察细胞数＝SCE／细胞

SCE ratio calculation：the SCE ratio can be calculated by dividing the cumulative number of exchanges by the number of observed cells，which is equal to the result obtained by dividing the number of SCE events by the number of cells.

（六）注意事项　Notes

（1）BrdU 溶液最好现用现配，一次用不完，必须 4℃避光保存。

The BrdU solution is preferably used fresh. If it is not used，it must be stored at 4℃ in the dark.

（2）BrdU 是强的致突变剂，使用浓度不宜太高，在每毫升含 25 mg 左右的剂量下不影响细胞增殖。外周血培养 24 h 后加入均可。

BrdU is a strong mutagen and its concentration is not too high. Cell proliferation is not affected at a dose of about 25 mg/ml. It can be added after 24 hours of peripheral blood culture.

（3）用紫外线照射诱发姐妹染色单体分化时，如紫外灯功率大，照射时间应相应减少。一般在 20 W 的紫外灯距标本距离应在 6 cm 左右；如果在 15 W 紫外线灯照射时距离标本应在 4 cm 左右。温度要控制在 50～60℃(冬天最好是 55～60℃)，但不应超过 60℃。如果时间过长或温度过高都易造成染色体肿胀。

During the differentiation of sister chromatids exchange induced by ultraviolet radiation, the irradiation time should be reduced correspondingly when the ultraviolet lamp power is high. Generally, the distance between the UV lamp and the specimen at 20 W should be about 6 cm. If the lamp is 15 W, the distance should be about 4 cm. The temperature should be controlled at 50 to 60℃, and preferably 55 to 60℃ in winter. An irradiation time that is too long or a temperature that is too high can easily cause chromosome swelling.

第四节 ◉ 小鼠骨髓嗜多染红细胞微核检测
Micronucleus test in mouse bone marrow polychromatic erythrocyte

微核(micronucleus)是游离于细胞质中的核物质小体,一般为主核的 1/4～1/3。微核是染色体畸变的一种特殊表现形式,是细胞分裂后期滞留的染色体断片或整条染色体在子代细胞分裂间期的细胞质中形成的游离团块物。由于染色体受化学诱变剂和辐射损伤而断裂成一些无着丝粒的染色体断片或纺锤体受到某些毒物作用而损伤,当细胞进入分裂后期时,染色体不受纺锤丝牵引而滞留在赤道板附近。在末期以后,单独形成一个或几个规则的次核,包含在子细胞的胞质内,由于比主核小得多,故称微核。微核同主核一样,是由 DNA 物质所组成。现已证实,微核率同外界作用因子的剂量呈线性正比关系。因此,微核检测技术已广泛应用在辐射防护、损伤,化学诱变剂研究和新药、保健食品的毒理实验中。

Micronuclei are small nuclear bodies that are dissociated from the cytoplasm and are a type of special manifestation of chromosomal aberrations. Micronuclei are often produced by the action of cells through radiation or chemical drugs, and are usually 1/4 to 1/3 of the main nucleus. Similar to the main nucleus, micronuclei are made up of DNA materials. It has been confirmed that the micronucleus formation rate is linearly proportional to the dose of the external action factor. Therefore, micronucleus test has been widely used in radiation protection, chemical mutagen research, and toxicological experiments of new drugs and health foods.

一、概述 Overview

微核的产生与染色体和 DNA 损伤有较大关系,常将微核的检出率作为 DNA 损伤的一种指标。微核检测(micronucleus test,MNT)方法可分成两大类。一类是从外周血中分离淋巴细胞,常规涂片即可,称直接法。该法制作简便、快速,适用于大面积的人群普查,但检出率低,敏感性较差,在精准反映染色体损伤方面一直有质疑。另一类是培养法,即将细胞经体外培养后再制片。该法检出率高,敏感性较强,而且制备的标本胞质完整、染色清晰。

微核的形成需要经过一次细胞分裂。有丝分裂阻断法微核检测技术是利用一定浓度的细胞松弛素 B 阻断淋巴细胞细胞质的分裂而不影响细胞核的分裂,即在淋巴细胞培养过程中加入细胞松弛素 B,使经过一次分裂的淋巴细胞呈双核,选择这部分细胞进行微核计数可以提高实验的敏感性。同时也成为检测致突变、致癌、致畸物质对机体遗传效应的一种重要手段。

微核技术与其他技术结合,实验方法日趋完善,试验选材范围越来越广,如小鼠、大鼠、中国仓鼠、猕猴、豚鼠等。各种实验动物中,小鼠价格便宜,骨髓中干扰因素少,是微核试验的常用动物。

The generation of micronucleus has a strong relationship with chromosome and DNA damage, and the detection rate of micronucleus is often used as an indicator of DNA damage. Micronucleus test (MNT) methods can be divided into two categories. One is the separation of lymphocytes from peripheral blood followed by conventional smear. This is called the direct method. The other type is the culture method, which consists in the preparation of cells in *in vitro* culture. The detection ratio of the culture method is high and it has strong sensitivity. Moreover, the prepared samples have a complete cytoplasm and clear staining. The formation of micronucleus requires a cell division. The mitotic blockade micronucleus detection technique uses a specific concentration of cytochalasin B to block the cytoplasmic division of lymphocytes without affecting the division of the nucleus. This method is an important means to detect the genetic effects of mutagenic, carcinogenic, and teratogenic substances on the body, and the mouse is a common model used for micronucleus testing.

二、骨髓微核试验　Micronucleus test in bone marrow

由于红细胞在成熟之前最后一次分裂后数小时可将主核排出,仍保留微核于嗜多染红细胞(polychromatic erythrocyte, PCE)中,因此通常计数嗜多染红细胞中的微核。微核经 Giemsa 染色后色泽鲜红,胞质内含有核糖体,被染成淡灰蓝色,微核,与胞质形成鲜明的对比,易于鉴别。

As the nucleus can be excreted in a few hours after the last division of the red blood cells before maturity, and because micronuclei remain in the polychromatic erythrocyte (PCE), the micronuclei in the PCE are usually counted. The micronucleus is bright red after Giemsa staining, and the cytoplasm contains ribosomes, which are dyed into a light-gray blue. micronucleus, thus being in sharp contrast with the cytoplasm and easily identifiable.

骨髓中嗜多染红细胞充足,微核容易辨认,自发率低,因此首选。而环磷酰胺因具有显著的诱变作用,常被用作骨髓微核试验的阳性对照物。除此之外,X 线、顺铂等也常用作阳性对照物或诱导剂。

The bone marrow has the advantages of the PCE, easy identification of micronuclei, and low spontaneous rate. Therefore, the bone marrow is the first choice for micronucleus experiments. Cyclophosphamide is often used as a positive control in bone marrow micronucleus tests because of its significant mutagenic effects.

(一) 仪器与试剂　Required equipment and reagents

胎牛血清、Giemsa 染液、PBS(pH 6.8)、甲醇、环磷酰胺、离心机、离心管、显微镜。

Fetal Bovine Serum (FBS), Giemsa staining solution, PBS (pH 6.8), methanol, cyclophosphamide, centrifuge, centrifuge tube, microscope.

（二）操作步骤 Protocols

（1）染毒：选取 2～3 月龄、体质量 18～22 g 的健康小鼠。小鼠腹腔注射一定量的化学物质及环磷酰胺（40 mg/kg）。

Intraperitoneally inject in mice aged 2 to 3 months and weighing 18 to 22 g with a certain amount of chemical agent and cyclophosphamide at 40 mg/kg of body weight.

（2）取材：以颈椎脱臼法处死小鼠，取两腿股骨，剔净肌肉，擦去附着在上面的血污，剪取两端股骨头，暴露骨髓腔，用注射器吸取 1 ml 胎牛血清，将注射器针头插入骨髓腔上段冲洗，用试管接收冲洗液，即成骨髓细胞悬液。

Sacrifice the mice by cervical dislocation. Remove the muscles from the two legs and collect the femurs. Cut the femoral heads at both ends and aspirate 1 ml of FBS into a syringe, to rinse the bone marrow cavity and collect a bone marrow cell suspension.

（3）离心：1 000 r/min 离心 5 min，弃大部分上清液，留少许液体，用毛细吸管将细胞团块轻轻吹打均匀。

Centrifuge at 1 000 r/min for 5 minutes and discard most of the supernatant. Leave a little liquid and gently pipette the cell mass evenly with a capillary pipette.

（4）涂片：滴 1 滴混匀后的液体于载玻片上，血常规涂片法涂片，自然干燥。

Drop the mixed liquid onto a slide, smear, and dry naturally.

（5）固定：玻片标本置于甲醇溶液中固定 10 min，晾干。

Fix the slide specimens in methanol solution for 10 minutes and air dry.

（6）染色：Giemsa 染液染色 10 min。自来水轻轻冲去多余染液，晾干，镜检。

Stain the slides with Giemsa staining solution for 10 minuters. Wash with water, air dry and observe under microscopy.

（7）观察：油镜下观察嗜多染红细胞的微核。典型的微核多为单个、圆形、边缘光滑整齐，偶尔呈肾形、马蹄形或环形，嗜色性与主核一致，直径通常为红细胞的 1/20～1/5。每张玻片标本计数 100～200 个嗜多染红细胞，按"‰"计算微核的出现率。微核计数以"细胞"为单位，即 1 个细胞中出现 2 个或 2 个以上微核时，只按"1"计算。

Observe the micronucleus of the PCE under a microscope using an oil-immersion lens. The micronuclei contained in the cells are mostly round or elliptical, and the edges are smooth and tidy. The color of micronucleus is consistent with the nucleus, which is purpler-red or blue-violet colored. One or more micronucleus can appear in one cell, and the diameter is usually 1/20 to 1/5 of the red blood cells. Each slide specimen contains 100 to 200 PCEs, and the occurrence rate of micronuclei is calculated according to "‰". The micronucleus count is in units of "cell", and when two or more micronuclei appear in one cell, only "1" is calculated.

（三）注意事项 Notes

（1）小鼠股骨较短、细，剪股骨头时，应尽量保持股骨中段的完整。

Because the mouse femur is short and thin, attempts should be made to keep the middle part of the femur intact.

（2）染液浓度、pH、染色时间等多种因素均可影响染色效果。例如，微核可被染成鲜红色、蓝紫色或紫红色，甚至在同一张标本上也会出现染色深浅不一致的现象。因此，计数前必须仔细观察 PCE 和成熟红细胞的差别，正确辨认。

Various factors, including dye concentration, pH, and dyeing time, can affect the dyeing effect. Before counting, the difference between PCE and mature red blood cells should be carefully observed and correctly identified.

（3）室温较低时，可适当延长染色时间。

When the room temperature is low, the dyeing time can be extended appropriately.

（4）正确掌握微核的形态特征，避免假阳性结果。PCE 中的 RNA 颗粒、含酸性多糖的颗粒以及一些附着的染料颗粒等经 Giemsa 染色后与微核颜色一致，易与微核混淆，应注意辨别。在实际应用中，如有必要，可采用其他方法重复试验，以排除假阳性。

Correctly grasp the morphological characteristics of the micronucleus and avoid false positives. Some RNA particles, acidic polysaccharide-containing particles, and attached dye particles in the PCE are consistent with the micronucleus after Giemsa staining, and are easily confused with micronuclei. In practical applications, other methods may be used to repeat the test and eliminate false positives, if necessary.

（四）预期实验结果及分析　Expected experimental results and analysis

1. 实验结果为阳性　Positive result

给药组与对照组微核率有明显的剂量反应关系并有显著性差异（$P < 0.01$）时，可认为是阳性试验结果。说明该化学物质能引起染色体断裂，是一种 DNA 断裂剂，但要排除假阳性结果。若统计学上有显著性差别，但无剂量反应关系时，则须进行重复试验，结果能重复者可确定为阳性。

If there is a significant dose-response relationship between the micronucleus rate of the drug-administered group and the control group, with a significant difference ($P < 0.01$), the test result is considered to be positive. If there is a significant difference but no dose-response relationship, trial repetition is required and the results can be scored as positive if they are repeatable.

2. 实验结果为阴性　Negative result

实验结果为阴性时，下结论要十分慎重。出现阴性结果的主要原因有以下几点。

When the experimental result is negative, the conclusion should be cautious. The main reasons for negative results are as follows.

（1）被筛选的化学物质不引起微核率增高。

The chemical substance being screened does not cause an increase in the micronucleus rate.

（2）制片时间不当：有些断裂剂能延迟红细胞的分裂和成熟，使出现微核的高峰时间推迟。因此，应根据细胞周期和不同物质的作用特点，确定取材时间。可先做预试验，一般为 30 h。

Improper production time: the time of the material should be determined according to the cell cycle and the characteristics of different substances，usually 30 hours.

（3）剂量过高或过低：各种化学物质的理化性质、体内代谢途径不同，应根据实验需要，根据药物的特点选择给药途径。例如，骨髓实验需短时间内达到有效浓度，应选用腹腔注射或口服用药。

Dosage is too high or too low：the route of administration should be chosen according to the needs of the experiment and the characteristics of the drug.

第五节 ◉ 荧光原位杂交
Fluorescence *in situ* hybridization

原位杂交(*in situ* hybridization，ISH)是一种在维持组织、细胞或染色体固有形态结构的基础上对其内部核苷酸序列进行特异检测及定位的分子生物学手段。ISH 的原理是将特殊标记或修饰的核苷酸探针与已固定的组织、细胞或染色体中的 DNA 或 RNA 杂交，并通过分析探针在被检对象中的显示状况，以完成目的核苷酸序列检测或定位。

早期的 ISH 技术是以放射性同位素标记探针和放射自显影技术为基本手段。由于放射性同位素标记法具有一定的危险性，且操作烦琐，而逐渐被荧光法、酶沉淀法或发色团检测等方法所取代。荧光原位杂交(fluorescence *in situ* hybridization，FISH)技术即是一种应用非放射性荧光物质依靠核酸探针杂交原理在核中或染色体上显示 DNA 序列位置的方法。

FISH 技术的优点在于：①探针稳定、操作安全、快速、特异性高；②多色 FISH 可以在同一核中显示不同的颜色，从而同时检测两种或多种序列。目前，已可用 5 种荧光素显示 23 种颜色来代表 23 对染色体，从而使核型分析直观简单；③FISH 也可用于间期细胞核内 DNA 的三维结构的显示；④反向染色体涂染可以精准确、客观地辨别新生染色体的来源；⑤微矩阵(microarray)技术和组织芯片技术使得一次性检测几百个基因或几百个组织成为可能，加快了检测的速度。

In situ hybridization (ISH) is a molecular biological method for the specific detection and localization of its internal nucleotide sequence based on the maintenance of the inherent morphological structure of tissues，cells or chromosomes. Fluorescence *in situ* hybridization (FISH) involves incubating lightly fixed thin sections of tissues or permeabilized cells mounted on glass slides with fluorescently labeled nucleic acid probes of known sequence or origin under conditions that allow specific binding to complementary sequences in DNA or RNA molecules in the samples. FISH is widely used in clinical testing，for example for the diagnosis of genetic diseases，analysis of viral infections，characterization of tumors and prenatal diagnosis，and is also an important tool in basic medical research and medical education.

一、FISH 常见类型　Types of FISH

（一）原位杂交显带技术　*In situ* hybridization banding
为了准确定位原位杂交部位所处染色体及其区带，染色体必须显带，但杂交与显带过程会相互影响。在人类短重复序列中存在 *Alu* 家族，片段长约 300 bp，在基因组中重复约 9 000 000 次。*Alu* – PCR 法是以 *Alu* 序列作为引物扩增 *Alu* 间的 DNA；由于 *Alu* 序列在基因组中分布不均，只有在致密区可以扩增出产物。以产物制备探针，通过杂交可以在染色体上形成类似 R 带的荧光带型。以不同的荧光物质标记目的探针与 *Alu* – PCR 探针，将可在染色体上同时显示杂交信号和染色体带型，这种荧光原位杂交技术称为原位杂交显带技术（*in situ* hybridization banding，ISHB）。

To locate accurately the chromosomes and their regions in the *in situ* hybridization site，the chromosomes must be banded，but the hybridization and banding processes will affect each other. The *Alu* family is present in human short repeats，with fragments of about 300 bp and repeats of about 9 000 000 units in the genome. The *Alu* – PCR method uses the *Alu* sequence as a primer to amplify the DNA. As the *Alu* sequence is unevenly distributed in the genome，the product can be amplified only in the dense region. The probe is prepared using the product，and an R-band-like fluorescent band pattern can be obtained on the chromosome by hybridization. The labelling of the target probe and the *Alu* – PCR probe with different fluorescent substances will display the hybridization signal and chromosome band type on the chromosome simultaneously. This FISH technique is called *in situ* hybridization banding （ISHB）.

（二）多色荧光原位杂交　Multicolor fluorescence *in situ* hybridization

利用不同颜色的荧光素标记不同的探针，同时对一张制片进行杂交，从而对不同的靶 DNA 同时进行定位和分析，并能对不同探针在染色体上的位置进行排序，形成多色 FISH （multicolor fluorescence *in situ* hybridization，M – FISH）。包括组合标记 FISH、比例标记 FISH，以及多色染色体涂色等。

Different probes are labelled with different colors of fluorescein and simultaneously hybridized to one slide. Using this method，different target DNAs are localized and analyzed，and the positions of different probes on the chromosome can be sorted to form multicolor fluorescence *in situ* hybridization （M – FISH）. These include combinatorial FISH，ratio-labelling FISH，and multicolor chromosome painting.

（三）比较基因组原位杂交　Comparative genomic hybridization

比较基因组原位杂交（comparative genomic hybridization，CGH）是一种改进的 FISH，通过对待检测的 DNA（如肿瘤细胞 DNA）和相应的正常细胞 DNA 进行不同颜色的标记（如肿瘤细胞 DNA 标记为红色，正常细胞 DNA 标记为绿色），同时与正常细胞的中期染色体进行杂交，然后根据两种探针荧光信号的强度差异判断待测与对照基因组 DNA 序列的拷贝数之比，找出待测基因组中的 DNA 扩增和缺失等变异，并描绘出相应的 CGH 核型图。

Comparative genomic hybridization （CGH） is an improved FISH that performs different color labelling of the DNA to be detected and the corresponding normal cellular DNA，and simultaneously hybridizes with the metaphase chromosome of normal cells. Subsequently，according to the difference in intensity of the two probe fluorescence signals，the ratio of the copy number of the test and the control genomic DNA sequences is determined. Mutations such as DNA amplification and deletion in the genome to be tested are detected and the corresponding CGH karyotype map is drawn.

（四）DNA 纤维 FISH　DNA fiber FISH

DNA 纤维 FISH(DNA fiber FISH)是一种应用各种不同的方法将细胞中的 DNA 在载玻片上制备出 DNA 纤维,用不同颜色荧光物质的探针与之杂交,并在荧光显微镜下观察结果以及进行分析的技术。与其他 FISH 相比,DNA 纤维 FISH 主要有如下优点:①高分辨率和定量分析,分辨率可达 1～500 kb;②模板要求不高,各种方式制备的线性 DNA 分子均可使用;③DNA 需要量较少;⑤灵敏度高。但也存在一些固有的缺点:①DNA 纤维的随机断裂可能导致同一探针的信号长度不一致;②DNA 纤维伸展的程度不一,导致不同荧光相互干扰,影响定量分析;③结果不能判断探针究竟具体位于哪条染色体上;④以同源的串联重复 DNA 序列为探针,杂交后在 DNA 纤维上散在分布的重复序列会产生杂交的信号不连续等。

DNA 纤维 FISH 在遗传学上具有广泛的应用,其不仅应用于精准作图和辅助基因克隆,而且也可定量分析不同克隆之间的排列顺序及重叠程度;定量检测染色体重排和缺失等异常;分析靶序列的拷贝数;决定基因之间的物理距离及其 $5'{\to}3'$ 定向;测量 DNA 座位的长度等。

DNA fiber FISH is a technique in which DNA fibers are prepared by various methods, hybridized with probes of fluorescent substances of different colors, and observed under a fluorescence microscope and analyzed. DNA fiber FISH has a wide range of applications in genetics, not only for accurate mapping and auxiliary gene cloning, but also for quantitative analysis of the order and overlap between different clones.

二、FISH 的基本程序　Basic steps of FISH

（一）样本制备　Sample preparation

用于 FISH 的样本可以来自于常规的血涂片、常规方法制备染色体玻片以及石蜡或冷冻切片等。为降低本底,杂交前可用 RNA 酶和蛋白酶 K 消化处理标本,然后再将玻片在 70% 甲酰胺中热处理一定时间,使 DNA 变性,最后于冷无水乙醇中退火,风干备用。

Samples for FISH can be obtained from conventional blood smears, chromosome slides, and paraffin or frozen sections. To reduce the background, the samples can be digested with RNase and proteinase K before hybridization, and then the slides are heat treated in 70% formamide for a certain period, to denature the DNA. This is followed by annealing in cold absolute ethanol and air drying for later use.

（二）探针　Probes

FISH 探针包括双链 DNA、单链 DNA、RNA 和合成的寡聚核苷酸探针。DNA 探针可分为四类:①基因组探针,多用于区分种间染色体或染色体区域的基因组 DNA 序列;②重复序列探针,其目标序列通常是染色体上不同部位的串联高度重复序列;能够在某一条染色体的着丝粒区或异染色质区产生致密的杂交带;③染色体文库探针(又称涂染探针),通常是用流式细胞仪从染色体悬液中分离出染色体,或对分带中期染色体进行不同程度的微切割

(microdissection)，再经分子克隆或 PCR 扩增制备染色体特异性探针，主要是针对染色体或染色体特异区进行杂交，用于检测分裂细胞中的染色体结构畸变和标记染色体；④单一序列探针，其片段一般比较长，必须插入到粘粒、噬菌体或酵母人工染色体（yeast artificial chromosomes，YAC)中进行扩增，主要用于单拷贝基因家族的检测定位。

探针标记分为直接标记和间接标记。直接标记就是将荧光素直接与探针相连。间接标记法是先在探针上接一半抗原，再用能同半抗原特异结合的带荧光标记的蛋白对其进行检测。标记方法多用缺口平移、随机引物标记和 PCR 扩增法。

FISH probes include double-stranded DNA, single-stranded DNA, RNA, and synthetic oligonucleotide probes. DNA probes can be divided into four categories: ① genomic probes. ② repetitive sequence probes. ③ chromosome library probes (also known as spread probes). ④ single-sequence probes.

Probe markers are divided into direct and indirect labels. Direct labelling is the direct attachment of fluorescein to the probe. Indirect labelling involves first the detection of half of the antigens on the probe, followed by its detection using a fluorescently labelled protein that specifically binds to the hapten. The labelling method mostly uses nick translation, random primer labelling, and PCR amplification.

（三）杂交　Hybridization

把变性后的探针加到处理后的玻片上，37℃杂交 16～20 h，杂交完成后必须将游离的探针充分洗去。晾干后加适量的抗褪色液。

The denatured probe is applied to the treated slide and hybridized at 37℃ for 16 to 20 hours. After the hybridization, the free probe must be thoroughly washed away. After cooling, an appropriate amount of anti-fade solution is added.

（四）检测和显色　Detection and color development

检测方法包括直接荧光法和间接免疫荧光法。如用荧光染料直接标记探针，可直接置于荧光显微镜下观察；若探针是用一个半抗原标记的，则可通过间接免疫荧光法进行检测。用生物素标记的探针经常用 FITC(绿荧光)、德克萨斯红（Texas Red)或罗丹明（Rhodamine）(红荧光)标记的亲和素来显色观察；也可通过生物素化抗亲和素抗体夹层逐级放大信号进行检测，玻片还常用 PI、DAPI 等补染，以便在荧光显微镜下观察杂交信号的同时，能看到胞核及染色体结构。

The detection methods in this technique include direct fluorescence and indirect immunofluorescence. If the probe is directly labelled with a fluorescent dye, it can be directly observed under a fluorescence microscope. If the probe is labelled with a hapten, it can be detected by indirect immunofluorescence. Biotin-labelled probes are often visualized using FITC (green fluorescence) and Texas Red or rhodamine (red fluorescent)-labelled avidin, and can be amplified step-by-step using a biotinylated anti-avidin antibody. Slides are also commonly stained with propidium iodide (PI) to allow the observation of the hybridization signal under a fluorescence microscope together with the structure of the nucleus and chromosome.

三、FISH 的应用　Application of FISH

（一）在细胞遗传学中的应用　**Application in cytogenetics**

常规的染色体研究方法对于小片段易位、倒位、重复和缺失难以分析。FISH 技术不仅可以应用染色体涂色方法检测间期细胞靶染色体数目变化，而且可以确定易位、重复、缺失或插入等染色体重排类型，为畸变染色体来源和断裂点提供可靠依据，并可鉴定环状染色体、双随体、双着丝粒、额外小染色体以及其他标记染色体等。

Conventional chromosomal research methods are difficult to apply to small fragment translocations，inversions，duplications，and deletions. FISH technology can use the chromosome painting method to detect the change in chromosome number of interphase cells，and can determine the type of chromosome rearrangement. Thus，it may provide a reliable basis for the determination of the source and fracture point of the distorted chromosome. It is also possible to identify circular chromosomes，bisatellite dicentric extrapolated chromosomes，and other marker chromosomes.

（二）在基因定位和基因制图中的应用　**Application in gene location and gene mapping**

FISH 不仅可以以目的基因为探针，对中期的染色体进行杂交，确定该基因在染色体上的位置；而且可以用于动植物基因组结构的研究和 DNA 分子物理图谱的构建。FISH 的分辨率决定了 DNA 分子图谱的精准性和精密程度。以中期染色体为 DNA 载体建立起来的分子图谱称为染色体分子图谱。由于中期染色体经过复杂的折叠过程，将导致两个荧光探针间的分辨率保持在 1～3 Mb。应用细胞同步化技术制备的前期染色体可以将 FISH 的分辨率提高到 175 kb。DNA 纤维 FISH 可以进一步将分辨率提高到 1 kb，与常规分子生物学的限制性内切酶图谱相近，但它具有更快速、更直接、更简便的优点。高分辨率的 DNA 荧光原位杂交技术能够快速准确地得到探针序列间的顺序、方向和真实的物理距离。

FISH can use the target gene as a probe to hybridize to the metaphase chromosome and determine the position of the gene on the chromosome. Moreover，it can be used for the study of the genome structure of plants and animals，as well as the construction of DNA molecular physical maps. The resolution of FISH determines the accuracy and sophistication of the map of the DNA molecule. A molecular map established using a metaphase chromosome as a DNA vector is called a chromosome molecular map. Because of the complex folding process of the metaphase chromosome，the resolution between the two fluorescent probes will be kept between 1 and 3 Mb. Pre-chromosomes prepared using cell-synchronization techniques can increase the resolution of FISH to 175 kb. DNA fiber FISH can further increase the resolution to 1 kb and is similar to the restriction endonuclease map of conventional molecular biology. Compared to other methods，it has the advantages of being faster，simpler，and more direct. High-resolution DNA FISH is able to quickly and accurately obtain the sequence，orientation，and true physical distance between probe sequences.

(三)在基因疾病诊断中的应用 Application in genetic disease diagnosis

FISH 技术是人类疾病临床诊断的重要手段之一。现有的高分辨分析方法不能检测诸如 Duchenne/Becker 肌营养不良、Prader-Willi 综合征等存在微小染色体缺失的人类遗传病。FISH 技术可以通过探针杂交,直观地观察到正常染色体存在杂交信号,而存在缺失的染色体无杂交信号,从而诊断缺失的存在与否。在血液病的研究中,特异的融合基因探针可以快速检测致病基因的存在。例如,*ABL* 和 *BCR* 融合基因的 FISH 探针可以筛选 Ph 染色体阳性的患者;Y 特异性 DNA 探针可以有效地诊断 *SRY* 基因等。

The FISH technology is one of the important means of clinical diagnosis of human diseases. This technology can visually observe the presence of hybridization signals in normal chromosomes via probe hybridization, with no hybridization signal in the deleted chromosomes; therefore, the presence or absence of a deletion can be diagnosed using this method. Specific fusion gene probes can quickly detect the presence of disease-causing genes in the study of blood diseases.

四、基于染色体标本的 FISH 实验 FISH assay for chromosome specimens

(一)原理 Principle

在已制备好的染色体标本或血涂片上进行 FISH 实验,在核中或染色体上显示靶 DNA 序列位置。

Do FISH assay with chromosome specimen or blood smears.

(二)仪器与试剂 Required equipment and reagents

甲醇、乙醇、乙酸、标记探针(生物素标记探针或地高辛标记探针)、3 mol/L 乙酸钠、甲酰胺、变性液、杂交缓冲液(4×SSC,20%硫酸葡萄糖)、漂洗液 A(50%甲酰胺,2×SSC)、漂洗液 B(0.1×~1×SSC, pH 7.0)、漂洗液 C(4×SSC, 0.1%Tween20, pH 7.0)、漂洗液 D(2×SSC, 0.05%Tween20)、鲑精 DNA、磷酸钠、Tween20、BSA、检测液(5 μg/ml 荧光素偶联的亲和素或 6 μg/ml 罗丹明耦联的抗地高辛抗体)、DAPI、离心机、荧光显微镜、旋涡混匀器、移液器、恒温水浴锅、培养箱。

Methanol, ethanol, acetic acid, labelled probe (biotin-labelled probe or digoxigenin-labelled probe), 3 mol/L sodium acetate, formamide, denaturant solution (70% deionized formamide, 2× SSC, and 50 mmol/L sodium phosphate), hybridization buffer (4× SSC and 20% glucose sulfate), rinse A (50% formamide, 2× SSC), rinse B (0.1× to 1× SSC, pH 7.0), rinse C (4× SSC, 0.1% Tween 20, pH 7.0), rinse D (2× SSC, 0.05% Tween 20), salmon-sperm DNA, sodium phosphate, Tween 20, BSA, test solution (5 μg/ml fluorescein-conjugated avidin or 6 μg/ml rhodamine-conjugated anti-digoxigenin antibody), DAPI, centrifuge, fluorescence microscope, vortex mixer, pipette, constant-temperature water bath, incubator.

(三)操作步骤 Protocols

1. 探针混合与变性 Probe mixing and denaturation

(1) 混合 20~60 ng 标记探针 DNA 和 3~5 μg 鲑精 DNA。反应后体积少于 10 μl,可直

接冻干；若体积较大，可加 1/20 体积的 3 mol/L 乙酸钠和 2 倍体积 100% 乙醇沉淀 DNA。混匀并于 −70℃ 放置 30 min。随后 4℃、12 000 r/min 离心 10 min，弃上清液，沉淀物以 300 μl 70% 乙醇洗涤后在离心（同上），弃上清液，冻干。

Mix 20 to 60 ng of labelled probe DNA with 3 to 5 μg of salmon-sperm DNA. If the volume after the reaction is less than 10 μl, it can be directly lyophilized. If the volume is large, add 1/20 volumes of 3 mol/L sodium acetate and 2 volumes of 100% ethanol and mix at −70℃ for 30 minutes. Centrifuge at 12 000 r/min for 10 minutes at 4℃ and discard the supernatant. Wash the pellet with 300 μl of 70% ethanol, centrifuge again, discard the supernatant, and lyophilize the pellet.

（2）将 DNA 重悬于 5 μl 去离子的甲酰胺中，室温旋涡混匀 3 min。

Resuspend the DNA with 5 μl of deionized formamide and vortex at room temperature for 3 minutes.

（3）加入 5 μl 杂交缓冲液，旋涡混匀 5 min。

Add 5 μl of hybridization buffer and vortex for 5 minutes.

（4）将 DNA 探针 75℃ 变性 5 min。迅速置于冰上 5 min，备用。

Denature the DNA probe at 75℃ for 5 minutes and quickly place on ice for 5 minutes.

2. 样本处理 Sample processing

（1）染色体制备标本或血涂片在室温下依次用 70%、90%、100% 的乙醇脱水，各 5 min。晾干备用。

Dehydrate chromosomal preparation specimens or blood smears with 70%, 90%, and 100% ethanol at room temperature for 5 minutes each, and air dry for further use.

（2）变性前将载玻片置于 60℃ 烤箱内孵育，目的是防止变性液加至载玻片时温度降低。

Incubate the slides at 60℃.

（3）将变性液在水浴箱中加热至 70℃。

Heat the denaturant solution to 70℃ in a water bath.

（4）将预热的载玻片移至含变性液的玻片染色缸内 2 min。

Transfer the pre-heated slides to a Coplin jar containing denaturant solution and incubate for 2 minutes.

（5）立即将载玻片依次移入 70%、90% 和 100% 预冷的乙醇中，各 5 min。防止 DNA 复性。

Wash with 70%, 90%, and 100% pre-cooled ethanol for 5 minutes each, to prevent DNA renaturation.

（6）室温下空气干燥玻片。

Air dry the slides at room temperature.

3. 杂交 Hybridization

（1）将 10 μl 含变性探针的杂交混合液加至载玻片上变性的靶 DNA 上。

Add 10 μl of the hybridization mixture containing the denatured probe to the denatured target DNA on the slide.

(2) 在杂交液上盖上盖玻片,防止产生气泡。

Cover the hybridization solution with a cover slip to prevent air bubbles.

(3) 用橡胶泥将盖玻片四周封好,并置湿盒内 37℃温浴过夜。

Seal the coverslips using plasticine and place in a wet box at 37℃ overnight.

4. 检测 Detection

(1) 从湿盒内取出载玻片,除去橡胶泥。

Remove the slides from the wet box and remove the plasticine.

(2) 将载玻片置于 42℃预温的漂洗液 A 中,在恒温水浴摇床中振荡 10 min,并使盖玻片脱落。更换漂洗液 A 2 次,每次振荡 5 min。

Wash the slides with rinse A pre-warmed at 42℃ and shake for 10 minutes in a constant-temperature water bath shaker, to remove the coverslips. Replace rinse A twice, shaking for 5 minutes each time.

(3) 将载玻片移入 60℃预温的漂洗液 B,漂洗 5 min,更换漂洗液 B 2 次,每次 5 min。

Wash the slides with rinse B pre-warmed at 60℃ for 5 minutes, replace rinse B twice for 5 minutes each.

(4) 将载玻片取出,甩尽液体,加 200 μl 封闭液,盖上盖玻片,防止气泡产生,置于湿盒内,37℃温浴 30 min。

Take out the slides and drain the liquid. Add 200 μl of blocking solution and mount with coverslips, to prevent air bubbles. Place the slides in a wet box and incubate at 37℃ for 30 minutes.

(5) 移去盖玻片,除去多余液体,加 200 μl 检测液(5 μg/ml 荧光素耦联的亲和素或 6 μg/ml 罗丹明耦联的抗地高辛抗体,缓冲液为 1% BSA、4×SSC 和 0.1% Tween20),在 37℃湿盒内温浴 30 min。

Remove the coverslips and excess liquid. Add 200 μl of the test solution and immerse in a wet box at 37℃ for 30 minutes.

(6) 将载玻片置于漂洗液 C 中,42℃振荡漂洗 3 次,各 5 min。

Wash the slides with rinse C three times with shaking at 42℃ for 5 minutes each.

(7) 将载玻片置于复染液(2×SSC, 200 ng/ml DAPI)中,室温振荡 20 min。

Place the slides in counterstaining solution and shake at room temperature for 20 minutes.

(8) 载玻片在漂洗液 D(2×SSC, 0.05% Tween 20)中室温温育 2 min。

Incubate the slides in rinse D for 2 minutes at room temperature.

(9) 荧光显微镜下观察。

Observe under a fluorescence microscope.

(四) 注意事项 Notes

(1) 在探针的混合和变性中,杂交液甲酰胺浓度必须根据 DNA 探针的特点进行调整。提高甲酰胺浓度可以增加重复 DNA 探针杂交的特异信号。

During the mixing and denaturation of the probe, the concentration of formamide in the hybridization solution should be adjusted according to the characteristics of the DNA probe. Increasing the concentration of formamide can increase the specific signal of repeated DNA probe hybridization.

（2）变性时间。当变性不够充分时，杂交反应不能有效进行；变性过度，将引起染色体DAPI复染模糊不清，使染色体形态丧失。

Pay attention to the denaturation time. When the denaturation is insufficient，the hybridization reaction cannot be carried out efficiently. If the degeneration is excessive，it will cause the DAPI counterstaining to be blurred and the chromosome morphology will be lost.

（3）在检测的过程中，必须保持载玻片的湿润。

The slides must be kept moist during the test.

（4）从荧光素标记到制片结束，整个过程须在避光下完成。避免由于光照，导致荧光淬灭。

The entire process from fluorescein labelling to the end of the preparation must be performed in the dark. Avoid fluorescence quenching caused by light.

（李枚原）

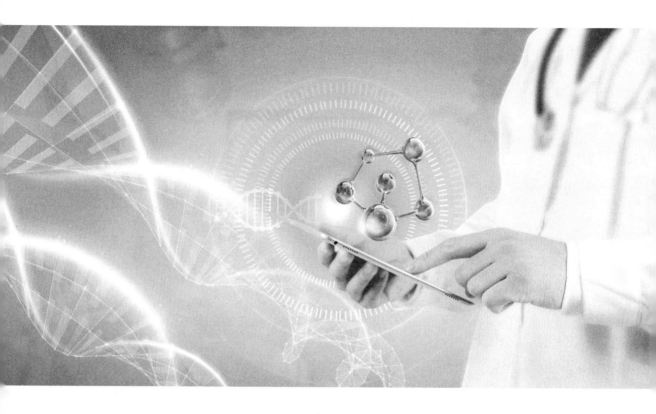

第三篇
遗传的家系和群体分析
Pedigree and population genetic analysis

第九章　遗传病的家系分析

Pedigree analysis in human genetic diseases

在人类遗传病的研究中，系谱是一个非常重要的研究工具。系谱依据个体间的亲缘关系绘制而成，向我们展示了一个家系中某种遗传病（或某个表型）的发病情况和遗传途径。系谱可以帮助我们分析个体的某个 DNA 片段是如何从父亲或（和）母亲那儿传递来的，既可以通过等位基因的序列差异直接判断，也可以通过 DNA 序列差异所引起的表型差异间接推断。

在系谱图中，箭头指明了该家系中第一个被发现的患者，称为先证者。从先证者入手，尽可能多地调查其亲属的患病情况，这有助于判断疾病是染色体疾病还是基因变异引起的疾病；是单基因还是多基因遗传；是显性还是隐性遗传；是常染色体还是性染色体遗传。事实上，系谱分析也是发现疾病、认识疾病的开始。在采集系谱时，重点应记录家族史、婚姻史和生育史。另外，对于收养、过继、近亲婚配和非婚生育等情况应予以注意。

Pedigrees are a key tool in human genetics. Pedigrees are a collection of related individuals that allow the observation of how segments of DNA are inherited by children from their parents. These DNA segments can be observed directly, as differences between homologous DNA sequences (alleles), or indirectly, in the form of phenotypes (such as diseases) that result from a specific underlying difference in sequence. Pedigrees illustrate the relationships among family members and show which family members are affected or unaffected by a genetic disease. Typically, an arrow denotes the proband, the first person in whom the disease is diagnosed in the pedigree.

第一节 ◉ 系谱分析
Pedigree analysis

系谱分析（pedigree analysis）是了解遗传病的一个常用的方法。其基本程序是先对某家系各成员出现的某种遗传病的情况进行详细的调查，再以特定的符号和格式绘制成反映家族各成员相互关系和发生情况的图解，然后根据孟德尔定律对各成员的表型和基因型进行分析。通过这样的分析，可以判断某种性状或遗传病是属于哪一种遗传病方式（单基因遗传、多基因遗传）。如果是单基因遗传，还可确定是显性、隐性或性连锁遗传。

Pedigree analysis is a general way to investigate genetic diseases. First, define the affection status of relatives in families; second, illustrate the relationships using pedigree notations; third, analyze the genotypes and phenotypes of family members by reference to Mendel's principles; last, clarify the inheritance pattern (monogenic or multifactorial inheritance; autosomal or sex-linked inheritance; dominant or recessive inheritance).

一、苯丙酮尿症(PKU)家系的系谱分析　Pedigree analysis of phenylketonuria (PKU)

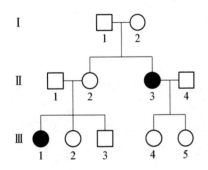

图 9 - 1　一个 PKU 家系系谱
Fig. 9 - 1　A PKU pedigree

苯丙酮尿症是一种氨基酸代谢异常疾病,常染色体隐性遗传。关于下列系谱(图 9 - 1),①哪些个体是肯定的 PKU 疾病基因携带者? ②Ⅲ 2 是疾病基因携带者的概率是多少? ③如果Ⅲ 3 和Ⅲ 4 结婚,他们第一个孩子是 PKU 患者的概率是多少? 第二个孩子是 PKU 患者的概率又是多少?

PKU is an autosomal recessive disease (a pedigree is shown in Fig. 9 - 1). ①Which individuals are heterozygous carriers? ② Determine the carrier probability of Ⅱ 2. ③If Ⅲ 3 and Ⅳ 4 get married, calculate the recurrence risks of their first and second children.

二、一例双生子家系系谱　A twins' pedigree

下列系谱(图 9 - 2),以生育双生子作为一个性状,其遗传方式是什么?
Determine the inheritance pattern of a twins' pedigree (Fig. 9 - 2).

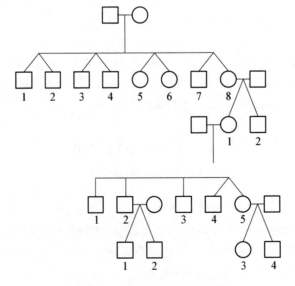

图 9 - 2　一例双生子家系系谱
Fig. 9 - 2　A twins' pedigree

三、1 例人类先天性耳聋的家系系谱　A congenital deafness pedigree

先天性耳聋呈常染色体隐性遗传,在以下系谱(图 9-3)中,Ⅲ4 和Ⅲ5 都是某一隐性突变的纯合子,他们婚后生有 4 个孩子,每个孩子的听力都是正常的。试解释之。

Congenital deafness is an autosomal recessive disease. In Fig. 9-3, individuals Ⅲ4 and Ⅲ5 have four normal offspring, please briefly explain why.

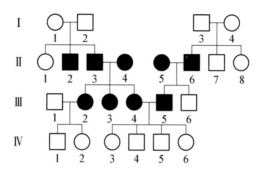

图 9-3　一个人类先天性耳聋的家系系谱
Fig. 9-3　A congenital deafness pedigree

四、一遗传病家系系谱分析　Pedigree analysis of a genetic disease

如果 a 是致病的隐性等位基因,相应的正常等位基因为 A,在以下系谱中(图 9-4):①母亲的基因型是什么?②父亲的基因型是什么?③孩子的基因型是什么?④疾病的遗传方式是什么?⑤子代中患者与正常孩子比例的理论值是多少?实际值和理论值是否存在差异(应用 Fisher's 精确检验)?

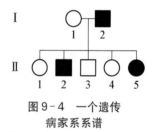

图 9-4　一个遗传病家系系谱
Fig. 9-4　Pedigree analysis of a genetic disease

Taking the lowercase letter "a" to represent a pathogenic recessive allele and the capital letter "A" for a normal allele, please answer the following questions (Fig. 9-4): ①Determine the genotype of Ⅰ1; ② Determine the genotype of Ⅰ2; ③Determine the genotype of Ⅱ1, Ⅱ2, Ⅱ3, Ⅱ4, and Ⅱ5; ④Determine the inheritance pattern of this disease; ⑤ Determine the theoretical ratio of affected/unaffected siblings; is there a significant difference between the theoretical ratio and the actual ratio (Fisher's exact test)?

第二节 ◉ Bayes 法在遗传咨询中的应用
Recurrence risks and Bayes' theorem

在预测单基因遗传病的发病风险时,如果不考虑患者家系中实际遗传情况,而仅按染色体分离与遗传方式计算,所获得的 1/2 或 1/4 的发病或再发风险概率,往往是不够准确的。

1963 年,Bayes 提出一种确认两种相斥事件相对概率的理论。当将这一理论应用于遗传咨询时,它不仅考虑该病的遗传规律和基因型,而且考虑到该患者家系中的具体发病情况。因此,应用 Bayes 定理能比较精准地推算出单基因遗传病的发病风险或再发风险。

Bayesian inference is a method in which Bayes' theorem is used. Bayesian inference takes advantage of the phenotypic information in a pedigree to evaluate the relative probability of two or more alternative genotypic possibilities and to assess the risk on the basis of that information.

一、应用 Bayes 定理计算时常用的几个概念　A few concepts about Bayes' theorem

(1) 前概率(prior probability)指所研究事件的概率,不考虑其他表型信息。提示一个个体是携带者的可能性(概率)是多少,不是携带者的可能性(概率)是多少。

Prior probability denotes the probability that an individual is a carrier before we account for the other phenotypic information.

(2) 条件概率(conditional probability)考虑到事件的真实性情况或特殊条件的概率,即一个个体如果是携带者,可根据该家系中遗传的参考信息,计算患有遗传病子女的概率和出生不患遗传病子女的概率。

We consider the phenotypic information by estimating the probability given that the individual is a carrier. Because this probability is conditional on the carrier status of the individual, it is termed a conditional probability.

(3) 联合概率(joint probability)即前概率与条件概率之乘积。

To obtain the probability of the co-occurrence of two events, we multiply the prior probability by the conditional probability, to derive a joint probability.

(4) 后概率(posterior probability)某一条件下的联合概率除以所有条件下的联合概率的和,也就是联合概率的相对概率。

The final step is to standardize the joint probabilities so that the two probabilities (i. e., being a carrier vs. not being a carrier) sum to 1. Subsequently, we simply divide the joint probability of the individual being a carrier by the sum of the two joint probabilities. This yields a posterior probability.

二、X 连锁隐性遗传病发病风险的估计　Recurrence risk assessment of an X-linked recessive disease

杜氏肌营养不良症(Duchenne muscular destrophy, DMD)是一种 X 连锁隐性遗传病,以男性发病为主,患儿的母亲为携带者。现以图 9-5 的一个 DMD 家系为例,利用 Bayes 定理计算Ⅳ1 将来发病风险如何。

如果按遗传规律计算,Ⅱ1、Ⅱ2 都已发病,表明这一家系中,致病突变不是新生突变(de novo mutation),而是隐性致病基因携带者Ⅰ1 传来,即他们的母亲Ⅰ1 为肯定携带者。因此,Ⅱ3 是携带者的概率为 1/2,Ⅲ5 是携带者的概率为 1/4,Ⅳ1 发病的风险则是 1/8。

但是,如按 Bayes 定理计算,则结果有所不同。首先计算Ⅱ3是携带者的概率(表9-1)。在不考虑其生育的情况下,她是携带者的前概率为1/2。但是,从系谱中寻找参考信息时可见,Ⅱ3已生出Ⅲ1、Ⅲ2、Ⅲ3、Ⅲ4 4个无病的儿子,这就是一个重要信息。因此,如果Ⅱ3是携带者,她连生 4 个儿子都无病的概率是 $1/2 \times 1/2 \times 1/2 \times 1/2 = 1/16$,如果Ⅱ3不是携带者,她连生 4 个儿子都无病的概率是1(即 16/16)。它们的前概率与条件概率相乘,即得出各自的联合概率,分别为 1/32 和 16/32。将两项联合概率作为分母,将每项联合概率作为分子,即可得出各自的后概率,分别为 1/17 和 16/17。由此表明,Ⅱ3是携带者的概率不是 1/2,而是降低为 1/17;相反,Ⅱ3不是携带者的概率也不是 1/2,而增高到 16/17。

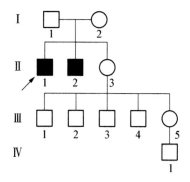

图9-5 一个 DMD 系谱
Fig. 9-5 A DMD pedigree

表9-1 Ⅱ3是($X^A X^a$)或不是($X^A X^A$)携带者的概率
Table 9-1 Carrier probability of Ⅱ3

概率	$X^A X^a$	$X^A X^A$
前概率	1/2	1/2
条件概率	1/16	16/16
联合概率	1/32	16/32
后概率	$(1/32) \div (17/32) = 1/17$	$(16/32) \div (17/32) = 16/17$

然后,再计算Ⅲ5是携带者概率。由于Ⅱ3是携带者的后概率为1/17,因此Ⅲ5的概率将为 $1/17 \times 1/2 = 1/34$,从而可以估计Ⅳ1的将来发病风险为 $1/34 \times 1/2 = 1/68$。

这表明按遗传规律计算和按 Bayes 法计算的Ⅳ1的发病风险,两个结果有较大的差异,由于 Bayes 定理考虑到了全面信息,所以其计算的结果更能反映家系子女发病的真实情况,预测的发病风险更为精准、可靠。

三、常染色体隐性遗传病发病风险估计 Recurrence risk assessment of an autosomal recessive disease

现以肝豆状核变性(hepatolenticular degeneration,HLD)为例,说明 Bayes 定理在常染色体隐性遗传病中的应用。

HLD是一种常染色体隐性遗传病。铜在细胞中的过量累积是细胞病变的原因,患者在发病的早期(细胞未发生不可逆的病理变化前)用排铜药治疗,可达到临床痊愈。然而,按遗传规律来测算 HLD 患者同胞的再发风险率(25%)的实际意义不大。临床生化检查(如血清铜、尿铜和血浆铜蓝蛋白的测定)在正常个体、HLD 基因携带者及 HLD 患者之间呈相互重叠,单独应用其中的某一指标都不能提高再发风险率评估的精准性,Bayes 定理可综合每个生化指标所提供的信息,从而提高再发风险率评估的精准性。

一家系如图9-6所示,先证者及兄妹均为HLD患者,现要评估先证者之弟Ⅱ4(目前临床正常)的再发风险率是多少?Ⅱ4现为7岁,根据发病年龄与发病风险关系曲线,知其发病风险率为0.766;血浆铜蓝蛋白为1.15 μmol/L,这一数值为正常个体、杂合子和(症状前)患者的条件概率分别为0.088、0.333和0.991(表9-2);血清铜为13.0 μmol/L,这一数值为正常个体、杂合子和(症状前)患者条件概率分别为0.290、0.533和0.030(表9-3);尿铜为1.68 μmol/24 h,这一数值为正常个体、杂合子和(症状前)患者的条件概率分别为0.093、0.147和0.923(表9-3)。另外,遗传指标酯酶D的分析显示Ⅱ4个体为正常个体、杂合子和(症状前)患者的条件概率为0.500、0.000和0.500(表9-3)。根据Bayes定理的计算公式计算出Ⅱ4个体为正常个体、杂合子和(症状前)患者的后概率,分别为0.101、0.000和0.899(表9-3),即Ⅱ4个体再发风险率约为90%,排除了其为杂合子的可能;该Ⅱ4经3年随防后证实为HLD患者,并立即进行了相应治疗,使症状得以控制,维持正常的学习和日常生活。

表9-2 HLD的3种性状在不同分组中所占的比例
Table 9-2 Proportion of three traits of HLD in the different groups

指标与分组	HLD的三种性状		
	正常个体	杂合体	患者
血浆铜蓝蛋白(μmol/L)			
<1.32	0.088(20)	0.033 3(24)	0.991(106)
1.32~2.64	0.836(189)	0.583(42)	0.009(1)
>2.64	0.075(17)	0.083(6)	0.000(0)
合计	1.000(n=226)	1.000(n=72)	1.000(n=107)
血清铜(μmol/L)			
<9.42	0.004(1)	0.233(14)	0.967(97)
9.42~15.7	0.290(65)	0.533(32)	0.030(3)
>15.7	0.705(158)	0.233(14)	0.010(1)
合计	1.000(n=224)	1.000(n=60)	1.000(n=101)
尿铜(μmol/24 h)			
<0.32	0.278(15)	0.147(5)	0.033(3)
0.32~1.28	0.630(34)	0.706(24)	0.044(4)
>1.28	0.093(5)	0.147(5)	0.923(84)
合计	1.000(n=54)	1.000(n=34)	1.000(n=91)

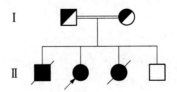

图9-6 一个HLD系谱
Fig. 9-6 An HLD pedigree

表 9-3 Ⅱ4 个体为正常个体、杂合子和(症状前)患者概率计算表

Table 9-3 Probability calculation of Ⅱ4

项 目	正常个体	杂合子	(症状前)患者
前概率	0.250	0.500	0.250
条件概率			
血浆铜蓝蛋白	0.088	0.333	0.991
血清铜	0.290	0.533	0.030
尿铜	0.093	0.147	0.923
酯酶 D	0.500	0.000	0.500
年龄/发病风险	1.000	1.000	0.766
联合概率	0.000 3	0.000 0	0.002 6
后概率	0.101	0.000	0.899

四、常染色体显性遗传病发病风险估计 Recurrence risk assessment of an autosomal dominant disease

一种常染色体显性遗传病的外显率为 60%，一个人的祖母患此病，他的父亲未患此病，他本人将来患此病的风险如何？试按 Bayes 法计算之。

(时文涛)

第十章　群体遗传分析相关方法

Analytical approaches of population genetics

群体遗传学是研究变异在人群中分布规律的遗传学分支学科,包括基因频率和基因型频率在群体内的变化和群体间的差异。群体遗传学的研究范畴既包括遗传因素(如突变和生殖因素),也包括环境因素(如选择和迁移),这两方面的因素共同决定了等位基因和基因型在群体中的分布及频率。

Population genetics is the quantitative study of the distribution of genetic variation in populations and of how the frequencies of genes and genotypes are maintained or change overtime both within and between populations. Population genetics is concerned both with genetic factors, such as mutation and reproduction, and with environmental factors, such as selection and migration, which together determine the frequency and distribution of alleles and genotypes in populations.

群体筛查是对群体中某种疾病患病情况的大规模调查,从而鉴定群体中个体的患病情况。群体筛查的目的不是为了精准地鉴定出患者,而是为了从人群中筛选出部分可能患病的个体进行更精准的诊断。而遗传筛查则是在群体中筛选携带致病变异的患者,或者筛选致病变异携带者的后代。过去人们主要依靠表型的测定来开展遗传筛查,比如某些酶的表达水平;DNA 相关技术的发展则让我们可以直接从基因型水平开展遗传病的诊断,本章将对一些比较重要的技术和研究方法进行简要的介绍。

Population screening is the large-scale testing of populations for disease in an effort to identify persons who probably have the disease and those who probably do not. Screening tests are not intended to provide definitive diagnoses; they are aimed at identifying a subset of population in whom further, more exact diagnostic tests should be carried out. Genetic screening is a population screening for genetic variants that can cause a disease in the person carrying the variant or in the descendants of the carrier. In the past, genetic screening usually relied on assays of disease phenotype. Advances in DNA technology have led to diagnosis at the level of the genotype.

第一节 ◎ 遗传平衡定律
Hardy-Weinberg equilibrium

群体遗传学的基础理论是 Hardy-Weinberg 定律,即遗传平衡定律。所谓遗传平衡定律,是指在特定条件下,应用一个简单的公式来计算群体内的基因型频率和表型频率,既可以通过基因型频率来推算基因频率,也可以通过基因频率来推算基因型频率。这个公式是由英国数学家 G. Hardy 和德国医生 W. Weinberg 1908 年提出和建立的。

The Hardy-Weinberg equilibrium is the basic concept of population genetics. The Hardy-Weinberg law was named for Godfrey Hardy, an English mathematician, and Wilhelm Weinberg, a German physician, who formulated this law in 1908. If a population under study ① is large, ② mating is random, ③ has no appreciable rate of mutation, ④ has no selection against any particular genotypes, and ⑤ has no immigration, we can use a simple mathematical equation to calculate genotype frequencies from allele frequencies.

一、基因频率的计算　Calculation of allele frequencies

按下述公式求出显性基因(p)的频率和隐性基因(q)的频率。

$$p = \frac{n_1 \times 2 + n_2}{N \times 2}$$

$$q = \frac{n_3 \times 2 + n_2}{N \times 2}$$

n_1:TT 基因型个体数;

n_2:Tt 基因型个体数;

n_3:tt 基因型个体数;

N:个体总人数。

二、基因型频率的计算　Calculation of genotype frequencies

用所求得的基因频率,按 Hardy-Weinberg 定律公式:

$$p^2 + 2pq + q^2 = 1$$

求出显性纯合子($TT = p^2$)、杂合子($Tt = 2pq$)及隐性纯合子($tt = q^2$)的基因型频率。

三、求各种基因型个体的理论值　Calculation of the theoretical number of individuals with different genotypes

将所求得的基因型频率与总人数相乘,即得群体中各基因型个体的预期理论人数。

四、卡方(χ²)检验　Chi-squared test

假设该群体是一个遗传平衡群体,检测各基因型的理论预期值与实际测得值之间的吻合程度进行验证。可用 χ^2 检验。公式如下:

$$\chi^2 = \sum \frac{(O-E)^2}{E} \quad O:实际观察值;E:为预期理论值$$

基因型个体数	TT	Tt	tt
实际观察值/O			
预期理论值/E			
χ^2			

求出的 χ^2 值若小于 $\chi^2_{0.05} = 3.84$, df$=1$(自由度$=1$),则说明预期理论值与实际观察值吻合,即该群体是一个遗传平衡群体。否则,该群体没有达到遗传平衡。

同理,可求出 ABO 血型的基因及基因型频率。

ABO 血型为复等位基因控制,达到遗传平衡时,各基因型频率满足于下式:

$$P^2 + q^2 + r^2 + 2pq + 2pr + 2qr = 1。(p = I^A; q = I^B; r = i)$$

第二节 ◎ 遗传病群体筛查的分子技术
Molecular tools for genetic screening

人们应用连锁分析和直接的突变检测来进行家系中遗传病的诊断,这些技术也可以应用到遗传病的群体筛查当中。针对很多致病基因已知的遗传病,人们已经开发出了 DNA 水平的直接检测方法。DNA 水平的检测现在不仅仅是传统非直接检测方法的补充,在很多情况下已经处于主导地位。

Linkage analysis and direct mutation diagnosis have been used for diagnostic testing within families, for prenatal diagnosis of genetic disorders, and more recently, for population genetic screening. In most cases, direct assays of disease-causing mutations have been developed. Genetic screening at the DNA level is now supplementing, and in many cases supplanting, tests based on phenotypic assays.

一、连锁分析　Linkage analysis

SNP 和 STR 等多态性位点作为基因组中的标记可被应用于连锁分析。如果某家系的连锁状态明确,我们可以对相关的多态位点进行基因分型,从而判定有患病风险的个体是从亲代遗传了包含致病突变的染色体区段还是正常染色体区段。因为连锁分析不涉及对致病突变的直接检测,所以是一种非直接检测方法。

DNA polymorphisms, such as SNPs or STRs, can be used as markers in linkage analysis. Once the linkage phase is known in a family, the marker locus can be assayed to determine whether an at-risk individual has inherited a chromosome segment that contains a disease-causing mutation or a homologous segment that contains a normal allele. Because this approach uses linked markers but does not involve the direct identification of the pathogenic mutations, it is a form of indirect diagnosis.

如图 10 - 1 所示是一个常染色体显性遗传乳腺癌家系。我们不需要确切知道图中所示的致病突变(pathogenic mutation)属于哪个基因,只需检测与之连锁的多态位点的基因型。针对一个多态标记的连锁分析显示第Ⅲ代女性从第Ⅱ代母亲遗传了编号为"1"的染色体,编号"1"染色体上携带致病基因。因此,这个第Ⅲ代的个体很可能在成年后罹患乳腺癌。

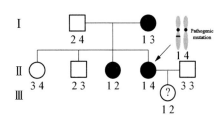

图 10 - 1　连锁分析举例
Fig. 10 - 1　An example of linkage analysis

在以往的工作中,人们已经应用连锁分析成功地诊断了多种遗传病。应用连锁分析时我们不需要知道明确的致病基因和基因表达产物,多态性标记仅提示某个体是否遗传了包含致病突变的染色体区段。随着直接检测方法的进步,连锁分析的应用逐渐减少,但对于致病突变不明确的家系,连锁分析还是有效的研究方法。

二、突变直接检测　Direct mutation analysis

对突变本身进行检测的方法叫直接检测,现在应用最为普遍。与连锁分析相比,直接检测不需要家系的信息,可以直接对每个个体的致病突变进行鉴定。另外,也不需要考虑序列重组所带来的影响。表 10 - 1 里总结了几种直接检测的方法,我们将在下一节对表中列出的部分方法进一步介绍。

Direct diagnosis, in which the pathogenic mutation itself is detected, has become the approach used most commonly in genetic diagnosis. Compared with indirect diagnosis, it has the advantages of not requiring family information (the mutation is viewed in each individual directly) and producing no error resulting from recombination. The various forms of direct diagnosis are summarized in Table 10 - 1 (the table is adapted from Nat Rev Genet, 2013, 14: 415 - 426).

表 10 - 1　突变直接检测方法
Table 10 - 1　Methods of direct genetic testing

方法 Method	单基因变异检 Single-gene Mutations	拷贝数变异 Copy Number Variants	单亲二倍体 Unipatental Disomy	重复次数变异 Repeat Expansions	应用举例 Examples of Applications
FISH		√			Williams syndrome; Prader-Willi syndrome

续 表

方法 Method	单基因 变异检 Single-gene Mutations	拷贝数变异 Copy Number Variants	单亲二倍体 Unipatental Disomy	重复次数变异 Repeat Expansions	应用举例 Examples of Applications
Array CGH		√	√		Intellectual disability or other conditions of unknown etiology
SNP microarrays	√	√			Cardiovascular disease risk; drug sensitivity
Allele-Specific oligonucleotide (ASO) hybridization	√			√	Sickle cell disease
Sanger DNA sequencing	√				Familial breast/ovarian cancer
Southern blot or MLPA		√		√	Fragile X syndrome
Targeted disease sequencing panel	√				Familial cardiomyopathy; Familial colorectal cancer
Whole-exome or whole-genome sequencing	√	√			Undiagnosed diseases of uncertain etiology

第三节 ◎ 基因组变异检测
Genomic variation detection

存在于不同个体基因组之间的变异,其范围可大可小,短至单个碱基(如 SNP,单个碱基的复制、缺失或插入),长至整条染色体(如非整倍体)。根据需检测变异的大小,人们建立了很多方法来满足不同的研究目的。但需要强调的是,无论采用哪一种方法的哪一篇论文,都无法百分之百地避免误差,如样本标记时的错误、数据生成时的误差等。

Variation between copies of the human genome exists over a wide range of physical scales, from single nucleotides to whole chromosomes. This method can be employed to detect and assay such variation and can be adapted to suit the scale of the variation to be detected. The armory of methods available currently is impressive; nevertheless, it is important to recognize that no method, and no published study, can ever be completely free from error.

一、DNA 样本的获取 Sources of DNA samples

无论要开展哪类基因组变异研究,都要有一定数量,来源于不同个体的 DNA 样本。能提取 DNA 的组织来源多种多样,从中提取的 DNA 量也有所不同。

As any study of human genetic variants requires DNA samples from several different individuals. There are several possible tissue sources differing in the amount of DNA that they yield and in other important aspects.

（一）血液　Blood

高通量测序中应用最广泛的是从人外周血提取的 DNA。静脉血容易采集，每 5 ml 可以提取 50～200 μg DNA。也可以通过 FTA 纸卡来保存干血点，从血点中提取 DNA。

（二）唾液或口腔细胞　Saliva or buccal cells

相对血液采集来说，收集唾液或口腔上皮细胞是无创的，也不需要专业的护士进行操作。但提取得到的 DNA 量相对较少（<1 μg）。

（三）精液　Semen

同样可以通过无创途径来采集。募集捐精者的过程比较敏感，所以在一般研究的起始阶段很少应用来源于精液的 DNA 样本。但如果想开展突变以及减数分裂过程中的 DNA 重组机制的研究，来源于精液的 DNA 样本就显得非常重要。

（四）毛发　Hair

从毛发中提取的 DNA 中有一部分会形成非常小的片段，即碎片化。但近几年在古 DNA（ancient DNA）的研究领域，人们发现在各种组织来源的 DNA 样本中，去除环境 DNA 对毛发样本的污染更容易，从而可以提取到更纯的古 DNA，用于进一步的测序。

（五）培养的细胞　Cultured cells

现有的培养细胞大多来源于两种组织：①皮肤活检样本中的成纤维细胞；②血液中的淋巴细胞。经 EB 病毒转染，淋巴细胞可被转化为永生化细胞系。比如在群体遗传学研究中常用到的 HapMap 和 1 000 genomes project 样本，都已建立了永生化的细胞系。需要注意的是，细胞系的传代过程常伴随新的基因组变异，如染色体的非整倍性改变、缺失、碱基替换和微卫星（microsatellite）重复次数改变等。

二、PCR、测序和人参考基因组　PCR，sequencing and the human reference sequence

关于 PCR 和测序，在前面的章节已经介绍，这里不再赘述。需要注意的是，PCR 的应用需要特异性引物，也就是说在开始实验之前，需要预先知道目的 DNA 片段的碱基序列。因此，除了 PCR 技术本身，人类参考基因组序列的测定也是非常关键的环节。PCR 产物的序列被测定后，还需要与参考基因组比对以鉴定变异。而测序技术在未来的发展可能会远超出人们的预期，将为群体遗传学研究提供强有力的技术支撑。

Because PCR relies on specific oligonucleotide primers, it requires prior knowledge of the sequence to be amplified. Therefore, other than the invention of PCR itself, the other key advance in human genetic diversity studies has been the determination of the reference sequence of human genome.

（一）针对目的区域或外显子组的测序　Targeted panels or exome sequencing

全基因组测序得到的数据量大，但成本也比较高。人们在开展遗传病致病突变检测的时候，常常只针对全外显子或每个个体的特定区域进行测序。如果仅针对特定区域进行测序，可以采用先 PCR 扩增，再进行二代测序的方法，不过这种方法比较耗时，目的区域也不能过长。例如，在一项研究中，针对 420 kb 的区域，进行了 124 个 PCR 扩增，这 420 kb 区域覆盖了与适应高海拔相关的基因。

　　另外一个途径是用 50～120 nt 长的探针(probe)来捕获目的区域,探针序列根据参考基因组设计,捕获的目的片段建库后测序。在全外显子组测序中,需要捕获约 1.6% 的基因组区(50 Mb),涵盖了几乎所有蛋白编码基因,还包含一部分侧翼序列(flanking sequence)及剪接位点(splice sites),绝大部分的遗传病致病位点都存在于上述区域内。Miller 综合征(OMIM 263750)是第一个应用外显子组测序发现致病基因的孟德尔式遗传病,相关论文发表于 2010 年。现在,外显子组测序已成为鉴定遗传病家系致病基因的常用手段。

(二) 测序数据的处理和解读　Sequencing data analysis

　　近几年,二代测序的实验成本逐渐降低,产生测序数据更加容易,数据的存储和计算处理成为研究者的主要工作。数据处理的复杂性主要源于两方面:①测序读长(reads)太短(100～150 bp);②较高的误差率。另外,一些插入或缺失(indels)也会给数据分析带来麻烦。图 10-2 展示了分析二代测序数据的生物信息学流程(bioinformatics pipeline)。

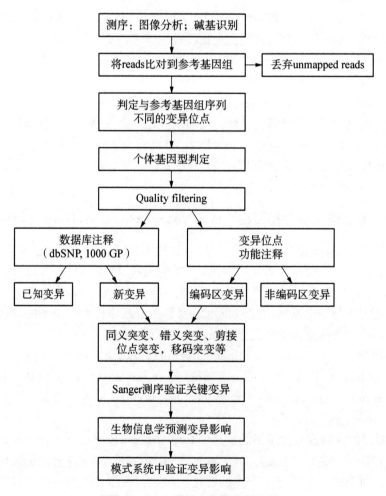

图 10-2　二代测序数据分析流程
Fig. 10-2　Next generation sequencing data analysis

数据分析的第一步就是把测序得到的短 reads 比对(mapping)到参考基因组上。如果测序得到的序列在参考基因组上没有同源序列,比对过程会不可避免地造成这些序列的丢失。为了避免序列丢失,可以对每个重测序数据进行重新组装(*de novo* assembly),但对很多结构复杂的基因组区域,组装则非常困难。例如,有人应用二代测序数据重新组装了两个人基因组,发现新组装的基因组比参考基因组短 16%,且丢失了参考基因组中 99% 的已知重复序列。

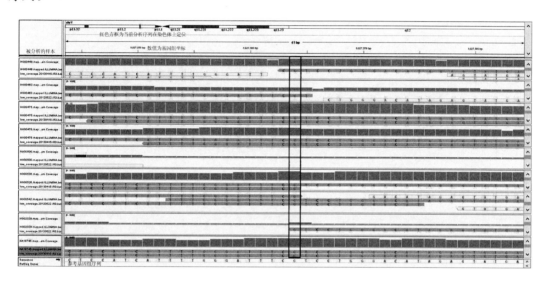

图 10-3　二代测序 reads 比对到参考基因组

Fig. 10-3　Mapping reads on a genomic sequence

　　应用 Integrative Genomics Viewer(IGV:www.broadinstitute.org/igv/;Robinson JT et al.(2011)Nat. Biotech. 29,24)将低覆盖度(low-coverage)的 reads 比对到人 Y 染色体上长 41 bp 的一段参考序列上(图 10-3)。图中每一个标记有碱基序列的灰色矩形代表一个 read,矩形的一端有箭头,代表了该 read 的方向。以黑色框内的碱基 G 为例,所有样本中的序列均与参考基因组相同,但可以观察到该碱基在不同样本中的测序深度不同。

　　如图所示,由于 NGS 是一种高通量测序技术,针对某个碱基,会有多个 reads 同时覆盖,某个碱基被覆盖的次数越多,也就意味着对该碱基的测序深度(read depth)越深,该碱基被正确读取的概率就越高。对于所有 NGS 数据,平均测序深度都是非常重要的指标。在千人基因组计划中,样本数量较多,样本的测序深度较低(2~6X),得到的数据覆盖了 85% 的参考基因组区,这些区域中 95% 的变异(人群中的频率>1%)被鉴定出来,这完全达成了初始研究目的。如果想让测序数据覆盖 95% 的参考基因组序列,平均测序深度则需要达到 50X。可以预见的是,随着技术和算法的进步,对测序深度的要求会有所降低。

(时文涛)

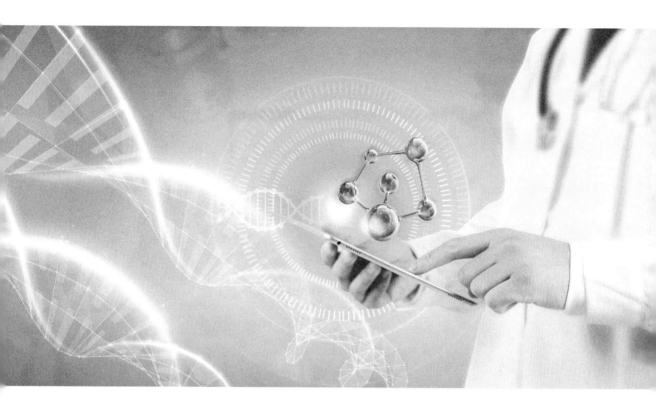

第四篇
细胞与医学遗传综合实验
Comprehensive projects on cell biology and medical genetics

第十一章 细胞生物学综合实验

Comprehensive projects on cell biology

现今的医学科学，需要基础与临床结合，强调转化医学，为将科研成果更好地应用于临床。这就对医生的科研思维能力有了更高的要求。因而对细胞生物学基本实验技术的了解、熟悉和掌握已经远远不能满足医学生的学习要求。综合实验的设计将有助于医学生科研思维能力的培养，综合运用所学知识独立分析问题、解决问题能力的提高。

包括人类在内的生物体都是由细胞组成的，细胞是生命的基本单位。正常生物体内细胞的增殖和死亡多处于动态平衡。平衡一旦被破坏，生物个体将会患病，衰老乃至死亡。以人为例，如果该死亡的细胞没有死亡，就可能导致细胞恶性增长，形成肿瘤；如果不该死亡的细胞过多地死亡，比如受艾滋病病毒的攻击，淋巴细胞大批死亡，人体的免疫能力受到破坏，将导致艾滋病发作。因而目前人类对于疾病的研究大多从细胞入手，进而进行动物实验和临床实验。体外培养的细胞是细胞生物学和分子生物学研究的一个常用材料。无论是细胞系，还是原代培养细胞均具备容易操作、易于观察等特点，同时又在一定程度上保存着与体内细胞相同的基本结构和功能，因而常被用来建立多种细胞损伤（紫外线、缺血、药物或某些化学物质等）或细胞保护模型（蛋白的上调或下调表达，药物等）。随后通过多项研究进行从现象的观察到机制的探讨，为各种生理病理现象乃至临床治疗提供一定的理论基础。

本章的综合实验将以培养细胞为实验对象，通过两个不同的实验案例，完成从现象观察到机制探讨的过程，提供实验设计的基本思路。首先对观察到的现象进行分析，通过文献回顾和已有的知识储备，考虑现象发生的可能原因，再设计实验进行证实，逐步深入，探讨现象产生的机制。为了便于实验教学的可操作性，本章实验设计尽可能选取易于实验教学操作的材料和方法。

The design of a comprehensive experiment will help medical students improve their scientific ability. The cell is the basic unit of life. Imbalance between cell proliferation and death leads to various diseases. Therefore, cultured cells are always used as a major tool in cellular and molecular biology. In this chapter, cultured cells will be used as the material, and a series experiments will be designed to clarify a specific issue. Students should analyze the observed phenomenon, perform a literature search based on the phenomenon, and provide a hypothesis. Subsequently, students should design the experiments that will be used to confirm the hypothesis and explore the mechanism of the phenomenon under study. Here, two experimental cases will be described in detail.

第一节 ◎ 细胞损伤综合实验
Comprehensive experiment of cell injury

恶性肿瘤已成为严重威胁人类健康的常见病和多发病,传统的恶性肿瘤治疗主要包括手术治疗和放、化疗。虽然随着生命科学的迅猛发展目前针对恶性肿瘤的治疗也有了长足的进步,但是由于肿瘤复发、耐药以及化疗药物不良反应严重等问题,恶性肿瘤的治疗还面临着很多瓶颈。随着对恶性肿瘤细胞增殖和死亡调控机制以及胞内信号转导通路的不断阐明,许多新的肿瘤治疗方法不断被研发和应用。其中包括了以关键蛋白为作用靶点进行的靶向药物研究。靶向药物会引发肿瘤细胞特异性死亡,并且很大限度地减少了毒副作用,对于特定的恶性肿瘤患者治疗优势明显。

Cancer is one of the most common causes of human death. The traditional cancer therapies include surgery, radiotherapy, and chemotherapy. With the remarkable progress in cancer research, many new cancer therapies have been developed, including targeted therapies. Targeted therapies can block specific proteins that participate in carcinogenesis with less side effects.

蛋白酪氨酸激酶(tyrosine kinase, TK)能催化多种底物的酪氨酸残基磷酸化,是信号转导通路中调节酶活性的重要蛋白。酪氨酸激酶功能失调,将导致其下游信号途径激活,调控细胞增殖的平衡被打破,最终导致肿瘤形成。因此,蛋白酪氨酸激酶也是目前抗肿瘤治疗的重要靶点。

Tyrosine kinases (TKs) control critical cellular activities by regulating signaling pathways. When overexpressed or activated by mutations, TKs can contribute to the development of cancers. Moreover, TKs have been the main targets of cancer therapy.

根据结构的不同,蛋白酪氨酸激酶可分为受体酪氨酸激酶和非受体酪氨酸激酶。表皮生长因子受体(epidermal growth factor receptor, EGFR)是一种受体酪氨酸激酶,定位于细胞膜上,是 EGFR 家族的一员,又名 ErbB1。包括肺癌在内的多种恶性肿瘤都存在 *EGFR* 的突变或表达增加。*EGFR* 突变或表达增加可能导致肿瘤细胞的增殖、肿瘤血管生成,加速肿瘤侵袭和转移及抑制肿瘤细胞凋亡等。而抑制 EGFR 酪氨酸激酶的活性将有效抑制肿瘤的生长。

Tyrosine kinases include receptor tyrosine kinases (RTKs) and non-receptor tyrosine kinases (nRTKs). The epidermal growth factor receptor (EGFR), also named ErbB1, is one of the epidermal growth factors in the RTK family. *EGFR* is overexpressed or mutated in many types of cancer, including lung cancer, and is the target of multiple cancer therapies.

肺癌是目前世界范围内发病率和病死率最高的恶性肿瘤,主要包括小细胞肺癌(small-cell lung carcinoma, SCLC)和非小细胞肺癌(non-small-cell lung carcinoma, NSCLC)。其中 NSCLC 又分为鳞状细胞癌、腺癌和大细胞癌。大约40%的肺癌都是腺癌。*EGFR* 突变在 NSCLC 中的腺癌患者中很常见。在亚洲人群中,具有 *EGFR* 突变的肿瘤患者约占 NSCLC

的 40%。靶向 EGFR 药物则成为了治疗肺癌的研发热点,包括作用于 EGFR 胞内区的小分子酪氨酸酶抑制剂(TKI)。TKI 主要通过竞争性结合 EGFR 的胞内段酪氨酸激酶的磷酸化位点,阻断其与 ATP 的相互作用,继而抑制 EGFR 的酪氨酸磷酸化及下游一系列信号通路,从而抑制肿瘤生长。

Lung cancer is the most common and fatal cancer worldwide. The two main types of lung cancer are small-cell lung carcinoma (SCLC) and non-small-cell lung carcinoma (NSCLC). NSCLC includes squamous cell carcinoma, adenocarcinoma, and large-cell carcinoma. About 40% of lung cancers are adenocarcinoma. Mutations in *EGFR* are common in NSCLC, particularly in tumors of adenocarcinoma. In Asia, the prevalence of *EGFR* mutation in NSCLC is about 40%. Tyrosine kinase inhibitors (TKIs) which compete with ATP for the ATP-binding site of PTK and reduce tyrosine kinase phosphorylation, thereby inhibiting cancer cell proliferation.

吉非替尼(Gefitinib)是第一代小分子酪氨酸酶抑制剂,可以可逆地和 ATP 竞争 EGFR 的 ATP 结合位点。研究发现,吉非替尼对具有 *EGFR* 激酶结构域突变的 NSCLC 具有非常显著的治疗效果,特别是对外显子 19 的小片段缺失和外显子 21L858R 的点突变。

Gefitinib is a type of TKI that reversibly competes with ATP at a critical ATP-binding site within the EGFR protein. Gefitinib induces dramatic clinical responses in NSCLC with activating mutations within the EGFR kinase domain, especially the exon 19 deletions and exon 21L858R mutation.

本综合实验将以第一代靶向药物吉非替尼为例,在细胞水平上探讨其对 *EGFR* 突变肺癌细胞的效果及可能机制,从而简要设计可供实验教学使用的细胞损伤综合实验。HCC827 细胞系是 *EGFR* 19 外显子缺失突变 NSCLC 细胞系,H358 细胞系则为 *EGFR* 野生型 NSCLC 细胞系。

This project will be an example of a research design. A series of experiments will be designed to explore the effect and possible mechanism of Gefitinib on *EGFR*-mutant lung cancer cells at the cellular level. The HCC827 cell line is an *EGFR* 19 exon deletion mutant NSCLC cell line, and the H358 cell line is an *EGFR* wild-type NSCLC cell line.

选用 HCC827 和 H358 细胞系进行实验,首先应明确 HCC827 和 H358 细胞系中 *EGFR* 的突变情况。提取两种细胞中的基因组 DNA(参见"真核细胞基因组 DNA 的提取"),随后设计针对 *EGFR* 基因的引物,通过 PCR 方法扩增出 *EGFR* 基因序列(参见"聚合酶链反应"),并进行测序(参见"基因测序技术")。根据细胞系特性,应该在 HCC827 细胞系中检测到 EGFR19 外显子缺失,而 H358 则含有野生型的 *EGFR*。

The mutation of *EGFR* should be identified in HCC827 and H358 cell lines. Genomic DNA should be extracted (See "Genomic DNA extraction from eukaryotic cells") and the *EGFR* gene amplified through PCR (See "Polymerase chain reaction") using specific primers. Subsequently, the *EGFR* gene from the two cell lines should be sequenced (See "Gene sequencing technology"). If HCC827 and H358 are the right cell lines, *EGFR* 19 exon deletion should be detected in the HCC827 cell line, while H358 should contain wild-type *EGFR*.

随后将细胞分为 4 组,HCC827 对照组、HCC827 处理组、H358 对照组和 H358 处理组。具体设计如下:相同数目的 HCC827 和 H358 细胞贴壁生长至对数生长期,对照组细胞继续给予正常培养基进行培养 24 h;处理组则给予含 0.2 μmol/L 吉非替尼的培养基培养 24 h。24 h 后首先对细胞的增殖活性进行检测,选用 CCK-8 法(参见"细胞增殖与活力")。比较吉非替尼处理 24 h 对两种细胞的增殖抑制情况。

The two cell lines will be divided into four groups, the HCC827 control group, HCC827 treatment group, H358 control group and H358 treatment group. HCC827 and H358 cells will be seeded onto culture plates or culture dishes. All media will be discarded when the cells enter the exponential phase. Then, in control groups (HCC827 control group and H358 control group), cells will be cultured with normal culture medium for 24 hours. In treatment groups (HCC827 treatment group and H358 treatment group), cells will be treated with 0.2 μmol/L Gefitinib in normal culture medium for 24 hours. To observe the effect of Gefitinib on the two cell lines, cell proliferation will be detected using CCK-8 (See "Cell proliferation and cell viability").

已有的研究表明,吉非替尼起作用的肺癌细胞几乎都存在 EFGR 激酶结构域的突变。而吉非替尼不起作用的肺癌细胞并不存在 EGFR 的突变。因而推测,吉非替尼能有效地抑制 HCC827 细胞增殖,而 H358 细胞则对吉非替尼有一定的耐受作用,即吉非替尼对 H358 的增殖抑制效果不明显。如果实际检测结果与预期相一致,则需要进一步思考,吉非替尼对 HCC827 的增殖抑制是通过怎样的机制产生的。

Nearly all Gefitinib-responsive lung cancers have somatic mutations within the EGFR kinase domain, whereas no mutations have been detected in non-responsive cases. Therefore, the predicted results of the CCK-8 assay will be that Gefitinib can significantly inhibit the proliferation of HCC827 cells, while Gefitinib has no effects on H358 cells. If the experimental results are consistent with the predictions, the possible underlying mechanism should be explored.

通过文献回顾,吉非替尼可能会诱导 EGFR 突变的肺癌细胞凋亡。因而选取 TUNEL 法(参见"细胞死亡")检测细胞凋亡情况,分组和处理时间点均与 CCK-8 实验相同。预期观察到的现象是 HCC827 处理组的细胞凋亡率明显高于 HCC827 对照组,提示吉非替尼可以诱导 HCC827 细胞凋亡。当获得的实际结果与预期结果相一致的时候,则需要探讨可能的机制。

Previous studies have shown that Gefitinib could induce apoptosis in lung cancer with *EGFR* mutation. Therefore, the TUNEL assay (See "Cell death") will be used to detect the apoptosis rate in the two cell lines after Gefitinib treatment. The predicted results are that the apoptosis rate in the HCC827 treatment group is significantly higher than that in the HCC827 control group. If the experimental results are consistent with the predictions, the possible underlying mechanism should be explored.

已有的研究表明突变 EGFRs 能够选择性的活化 Akt 及 STAT 信号通路,从而促进细胞存活。因此,可以通过免疫印迹的方法(参见"免疫印迹")检测吉非替尼作用于 HCC827 细胞后 Akt 和 STAT 信号通路的活化情况。预期 HCC827 处理组中 Akt 和 STAT 的磷酸化水平降低,提示吉非替尼能够抑制 Akt 和 STAT 信号通路的活化。如果实际检测结果与预期相一致,则需要进一步思考吉非替尼诱导 HCC827 细胞凋亡,进而抑制 HCC827 细胞增殖是否通过抑制 Akt 和 STAT 信号通路的活化。

Previous studies have shown that mutant EGFRs selectively activate Akt and the signal transduction and activator of transcription (STAT) signaling pathways, which promote cell survival. Therefore, the activation of the Akt and STAT signaling pathways should be detected through immunoblotting (See "Immunoblotting"). The predicted results are that the phosphonate of Akt and STAT are decreased after Gefitinib treatment. If the experimental results are consistent with the predictions, whether Gefitinib induce HCC827 cells apoptosis through the inhibition of Akt and STAT signaling pathways or not should be explored.

为此需要通过一系列实验活化 Akt 和 STAT 信号通路,如果活化的信号通路能够逆转吉非替尼对 HCC827 的凋亡诱导作用,则提示吉非替尼能通过抑制 Akt 和 STAT 的活化诱导的 HCC827 凋亡,进而抑制细胞增殖。

So if the activation of Akt and STAT signaling pathways can relatively resistant to apoptosis induced by Gefitinib, we can conclude that Gefitinib can induce HCC827 cells apoptosis through the inhibition of Akt and STAT signaling pathways.

技术路线图如图 11-1。

Technical route (Fig. 11-1).

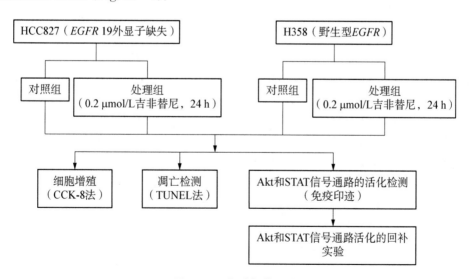

图 11-1　细胞损伤实验

Fig. 11-1　Experiment of cell injury

据此,设计一个关于细胞损伤的具体方案,并绘制技术路线图。

Base on this project, please design a new project about cell injury and draw the technical route.

第二节 ◎ 细胞保护综合实验
Comprehensive experiment of cell protection

缺血性疾病是危害人类健康的常见病，当缺血严重超出人体的代偿机制时，就会产生不可逆的细胞死亡，也是人类死亡的重要原因之一。体内缺血主要包括缺糖和缺氧两种损伤形式。其中葡萄糖是细胞内能量代谢的核心，也是一些神经退行性疾病如阿尔茨海默病、肌萎缩侧索硬化症的发病机制之一。

脑缺血是人体内常见的会导致严重后果的病理状态，缺血神经元损伤的机制日益受到人们的关注。人们在探讨缺血导致神经元损伤可能机制的同时，也在寻找更好的保护神经元的方法。谷氨酰胺是一种人体内的条件必需氨基酸，在体液中含量丰富，占总游离氨基酸的 61%，主要储存于脑和骨骼肌内。已有研究表明，谷氨酰胺能够保护细胞免受缺糖损伤的影响。

Ischemia means the interruption of blood supply, which leads to deprived oxygen and glucose. Cerebral ischemia, which can lead to neuronal cell death, is the most common cause of death worldwide. Researchers want to explore the mechanism of neuronal cell death caused by cerebral ischemia.

缺糖（glucose deprivation, GD）是缺血过程中的关键因素，探讨缺糖损伤对神经细胞的影响，将有助于从细胞水平上研究缺血过程中神经元损伤的可能机制。大鼠肾上腺嗜铬细胞瘤（rat adrenal pheochromocytoma, PC12）细胞能够合成并储存多巴胺和去甲肾上腺素等神经递质，是最常用的神经细胞模型。本实验拟探讨缺糖对神经细胞的损伤作用，以及谷氨酰胺对缺糖损伤细胞的保护作用，并对可能的机制进行研究。

Glucose deprivation is a key factor in ischemia, and the rat adrenal pheochromocytoma PC12 cell line is a classical neuronal cell model. Glutamine is an amino acid that has many essential functions in cells, including the protection of neurons. Therefore, the aim of this project is to observe the effect of glucose deprivation on PC12 cells and the protection afforded by glutamine in PC12 cells under glucose deprivation. Subsequently, a series experiments will be designed to explore the possible underlying mechanism.

选用 PC12 细胞进行相关实验研究，分为对照组（正常培养）、损伤组（缺糖培养）、保护组（缺糖培养的同时进行谷氨酰胺处理）。为方便实验教学的可行性，通过预实验选择某特定的时间点（如 24 h）和合适的谷氨酰胺浓度（如 2 mmol/L）进行相关指标的检测。具体设计如下：取相同数目的 PC12 细胞接种于培养板或培养皿，贴壁生长至对数生长期。弃去原有培养基后，对照组细胞继续给予正常培养基进行培养；损伤组则用无糖培养基替代正常培养基，在缺糖条件下继续培养；保护组是指在 PC12 细胞缺糖培养的同时给予 2 mmol/L 谷氨酰胺处理，3 组细胞同时培养 24 h 后进行不同指标的检测。为明确缺糖对神经细胞的损伤作用，以及谷氨酰胺对缺糖损伤细胞的保护作用，首先检测缺糖处理后以及谷氨酰胺干预后，PC12 细胞的增殖情况。本实验通过 CCK-8 法（参见"细胞增殖与活力"）检测三组细胞的增殖活性。

PC12 cells will be divided into three groups, the control group, injury group and protection group. PC12 cells will be seeded onto culture plates or culture dishes prior to treatment. When cells enter the exponential phase, all media will be discarded. In the control group, cells will be cultured with normal culture medium. In the injury group, cells will be cultured with glucose-deprived medium. Finally, in the protection group, cells will be cultured with 2 mmol/L glutamine in glucose-deprived medium. All cells will be incubated for an additional 24 hours before detection.

To assess the effect of glucose deprivation in PC12 cells and the protection afforded by glutamine in these cells under glucose deprivation, cell proliferation will be detected using CCK - 8 (See "Cell proliferation and cell viability").

根据已有的研究,推测缺糖将导致 PC12 细胞增殖活性降低,而谷氨酰胺可以抑制缺糖引起的细胞增殖活性降低。如果实际检测结果与预期相一致,则需要进一步思考,细胞增殖活性降低的可能原因。

Previous studies showed that PC12 cell proliferation was decreased after glucose withdrawal, and that glutamine can inhibit this decrease in cell proliferation. If the experimental results are consistent with the predictions, the underlying mechanism should be explored.

细胞死亡往往是细胞增殖活性降低的重要因素。细胞死亡的模式很多,包括"典型"的死亡形式(坏死、凋亡和自噬)和非典型细胞死亡(atypical cell death)。通过文献回顾,得知缺糖等应激因素可能会引起细胞凋亡,而谷氨酰胺可以抑制细胞的凋亡。那么,缺糖引发的 PC12 细胞增殖活性降低及谷氨酰胺介导的细胞保护作用是否与细胞凋亡有关,需要进一步的实验研究。

Cell death is a key cause of reduced cell proliferation. There are different types of cell death, including apoptosis, autophagy, necrosis, and some other atypical cell death. A previous study showed that glucose deprivation can induce cell apoptosis, and that glutamine can inhibit cell apoptosis. Whether the decreased PC12 cell proliferation is caused by apoptosis, and whether the apoptosis can be inhibited by glutamine warrants further elucidation.

选取适合实验教学的凋亡相关实验检测方法(参见"细胞死亡"),分组和处理时间点均与 CCK - 8 实验相同。预期观察到的现象是损伤组细胞凋亡率明显高于对照组和保护组,提示缺糖可以诱导 PC12 细胞凋亡,而谷氨酰胺可以抑制缺糖诱导的细胞凋亡。当获得的实际结果与预期结果相一致时,则需要探讨该现象发生的可能机制。

A suitable apoptosis assay will be selected for experimental teaching (See "Cell death"). PC12 cells will be divided into three groups. The predicted results are that the apoptosis rate of the injury group is significantly higher than that of the control group and the protection group. If the experimental results are consistent with the predictions, the underlying mechanism should be explored.

凋亡是多细胞生物体维持正常发育和正常稳态的关键。细胞外的凋亡诱导因子作用于靶细胞时,可以通过细胞内不同的信号转导通路,最终激活细胞死亡程序,导致细胞凋亡。细胞内存在着两条主要的凋亡相关通路:细胞表面死亡受体介导的"外源性凋亡通路"和由线粒体介导的"内源性凋亡通路"。其中内源性凋亡通路的核心细胞器是线粒体。细胞色素C(cytochrome C,Cyt C)和其他促凋亡因子从线粒体向胞质的释放是内源性凋亡通路中关键的控制因素。释放入胞质的 Cyt C 与凋亡酶激活因子(apoptotic protease activating factor 1,Apaf-1)结合形成复合体,进而使 Caspase-9 酶原活化,启动 Caspase 级联反应,触发凋亡程序。研究提示细胞在多种应激作用下往往会启动内源性凋亡通路,引发随后的细胞死亡。为此,可以通过检测 Cyt C 从线粒体释放入胞质的情况,以明确缺糖是否启动内源性凋亡通路。使用 Cyt C 抗体,通过免疫细胞化学的方法检测 3 组细胞中 Cyt C 在线粒体和胞质的分布情况[参见"免疫组织(细胞)化学技术"]。预期与对照组相比,损伤组可以观察到 Cyt C 从线粒体易位至胞质的现象,提示缺糖可以启动内源性凋亡通路;而保护组中 Cyt C 的易位现象并不明显,提示谷氨酰胺抑制了 Cyt C 从线粒体向胞质的释放。实际检测结果与预期相一致时,可以探讨 Cyt C 释放入胞质的上游调控机制。

Apoptosis is essential for the normal development and tissue homeostasis of all multicellular organisms. Two distinct pathways of apoptosis have been described, the death receptor pathway (the extrinsic apoptotic pathway) and the mitochondrial pathway (the intrinsic apoptotic pathway). Moreover, the release of cytochrome C(Cyt C) and other pro-apoptogenic factors from mitochondria into the cytosol is an important step in the intrinsic pathway of apoptosis. The released Cyt C binds to apoptotic protease activating factor 1 (Apaf-1) and caspase-9, which activate a series of caspases and induce cell apoptosis. Under various stresses, cells have the option of actively engaging in the intrinsic apoptotic pathway. Whether the apoptosis of PC12 cells induced by glucose deprivation occurs via the intrinsic apoptotic pathway, and whether glutamine plays a role in regulating the release of Cyt C warrant further exploration. The release of Cyt C from mitochondria into the cytosol will be measured in three groups using immunofluorescence (See "Immunohistochemistry and immunocytochemistry"). If the experimental results are consistent with the predictions, the regulation of Cyt C release should be explored.

Bcl-2 家族成员是调节内源性凋亡通路的线粒体上游分子,可以通过控制 Cyt C 的释放影响凋亡的进程。Bax 是 Bcl-2 蛋白家族中的一个促凋亡蛋白。非应激细胞中 Bax 主要以单体的形式存在于胞质中,凋亡信号作用于细胞时可引起 Bax 构象的改变而活化,活化的 Bax 易位至线粒体的外膜发生寡聚化,促进了线粒体外膜的通透性转换孔的形成和开放,从而释放出 Cyt C 和凋亡诱导因子,激活内源性细胞凋亡途径。那么,缺糖诱导 Cyt C 从线粒体向胞质的释放以及谷氨酰胺对该过程的抑制,是否经由 Bax 的活化? 可以使用 Bax 构象改变特异性抗体(Bax6A7),通过免疫细胞化学方法检测 Bax 的活化和易位情况(参见"免疫组织(细胞)化学技术")。预期与对照组相比,可以在损伤组中观察到活化的 Bax 阳性细胞比例增高,而保护组中 Bax 阳性细胞比例较损伤组少。当实际检测结果与预期相一致时,需进一步探讨调控 Bax 活化的可能机制。

The release of Cyt C is regulated by a complex balance of pro-apoptotic and anti-apoptotic proteins of the Bcl-2 family. Previous studies have shown that the conformational change of Bax is an important factor in the regulation of Cyt C release. Bax is a monomeric and predominant cytosolic protein in unstressed cells. Apoptotic signals induce the Bax conformational change, leading to its translocation to the outer mitochondrial membrane, where its oligomerization causes membrane permeabilization and Cyt C release.

Immunofluorescence (See "Immunohistochemistry and immunocytochemistry") will be used to detect the conformational change of Bax using a special Bax-conformation-specific antibody (Bax6A7). Bax6A7 only recognizes the form of Bax that is competent for membrane insertion. If the experimental results are consistent with the predictions, the regulation of the Bax conformational change should be explored.

已有的研究表明,多条信号转导通路可能参与了缺血诱导的神经细胞凋亡:磷脂酰肌醇 3 激酶(Phosphatidylinositol 3 kinase,PI3K)/Akt 途径和丝裂原活化蛋白激酶(mitogen-activated protein kinase,MAPK)途径中的胞外信号调节激酶(extracellular signal-regulated protein kinase,Erk)、应激活化蛋白激酶(stress-activated protein kinase,SAPK)和蛋白激酶 p38 所介导的信号转导通路。那么这些信号转导通路(Ras/Raf/MEK/ERK 通路、PI3K/AKT 通路等)的活化是否可以作用于 Bax 从而调控内源性凋亡通路? 可以通过特异性的通路抑制剂和免疫印迹(western blotting)技术探讨在缺糖条件下多个信号通路是否参与 Bax 活性的调控。

Previous studies have shown that many signaling pathways participate in the neuronal apoptosis induced by ischemia, such as PI3K/Akt and Ras/Raf/MEK/ERK. Whether these signaling pathways regulate the Bax conformational change induced by glucose deprivation, and whether glutamine regulates these signaling pathways warrant further investigation.

技术路线图如下:

Technical route：

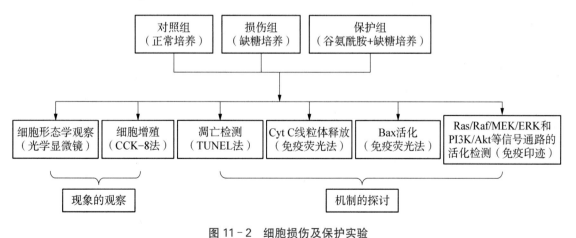

图 11 - 2　细胞损伤及保护实验

Fig. 11 - 2　Experiment of cell injury and protection

据此,设计一个关于细胞损伤与保护研究的具体方案,并绘制其他细胞损伤和保护的技术路线图。

Base on this project，please design a new project about cell injury and protection and draw the technical route.

（杨　玲）

第十二章 遗传病的诊断、分析与咨询实验

Diagnosis, analysis, and consultation on genetic diseases

病例一 Case 1

姓名:李× 性别:女 出生日期:1986 年 12 月 6 日

民族:汉 地址:江苏省××县××乡

就诊日期:2018 年 5 月

主诉:2015 年 8 月生育一男婴,出生时未觉异常,但吸吮能力较弱;生长速度比别的婴儿慢,3 个月时发现其尚不能抬头,2 岁时始能独立行走和说话,至今只能说简单词语,认知能力、辨别能力均较其他幼儿差。到当地卫生院就诊后认为该幼儿有严重的智力障碍,但未作进一步检查。目前,李×已怀孕 16 周,急需知道所怀胎儿是否正常。

Name: Li   Gender: Female   Date of Birth: December 6th, 1986

Address: ×× County, ×× Town, Jiangsu Province

Date of hospital visit: May 2018

Chief complaint: The patient had a baby boy in August of 2015. The baby seemed normal when he was born, but had dysthelasia. The baby grew more slowly than other infants, could not raise his head at 3 months of age, and started walking independently and talking at 2 years of age. His mental abilities (thinking, reasoning, and understanding) were poorer than those of normal children. The local hospital diagnosed mental retardation. The mother is currently pregnant again (16 weeks) and is anxious to learn if her unborn baby is healthy.

一、诊断 Diagnosis

(一) 患儿的诊断 Patient diagnosis

1. 病史与家族史采集 Medical history and family history review

患儿唐×,2005 年 8 月出生,病史见主诉;无家族史。

2. 症状与体征 Physical symptoms

特殊面容(眼距宽,外眼角上斜,鼻部低平,张口伸舌、流涎),肌张力低,双手均为通关手;严重智障;隐睾。

根据患儿的症状与体征,初步判断可能为 Down 综合征,须做染色体检查以确诊。

Physical Symptoms: Facial features (wild-span eye distance, flatter faces, especially the nose, and a tongue that sticks out of the mouth). A single deep crease across the center of the palm. Low muscle tone. Mental retardation. Retained testicle.

According to the symptoms and the physical characteristics, the child was suspected to have Down syndrome.

3. 染色体检查 Chromosome analysis

患儿外周静脉采血 2 ml,肝素抗凝,制备染色体标本(参加"人类染色体标本的制备"),G 显带(参见"染色体 G 显带技术")染色后镜检并通过染色体图像分析软件分析结果。

检查结果:患儿核型为 46,XY,+21

Chromosome analysis (See "Human chromosome preparation" and "G banding")

诊断:Down 综合征

李×已生一胎 Down 综合征患儿,再次生育 Down 综合征的再发风险升高,建议做产前诊断。

Chromosome karyotype:46,XY,+21

Diagnosis:The examination of the karyotype revealed that the child had Down syndrome. It was suggested that the mother undergo prenatal screening to estimate the chance of the fetus having Down syndrome.

(二)李×的产前诊断 Prenatal diagnosis

1. 病史 Medical history

两次妊娠史,已生育一 Down 综合征患儿,本次妊娠为第二次妊娠,目前孕 16 周,无明显早孕反应,孕前和怀孕后均无患病、服药和接触有害物质。在当地医院做产前检查均正常。

2. Down 综合征产前筛查 Prenatal screening

Down 综合征产前筛查(三联征产前筛查),检查时间为 14~20 周。检查血清中甲胎蛋白(AFP),血清绒毛膜促性腺激素(hCG),血清游离雌三醇(E_3)。

检查结果:AFP 15 ng/ml

hCG 4.62×10^3 IU/ml

E_3 17.7 mol/L

经计算机软件分析,Down 综合征高风险的切割值(cut off)>1:20,筛查显示李×为 Down 综合征高风险产妇。

三联征产前筛查显示了李×为高风险产妇,但三联征产前筛查存在 5% 的假阳性率,须做胎儿染色体检查确诊。目前,孕周 16 周适宜做羊水染色体检查(16~20 周)。

3. 胎儿染色体检查 Fetal examination

(1)无创染色体检查 Non-invasive prenatal testing of fetal chromosome:抽取孕妇外周血 10 ml,肝素抗凝。采血后立即缓慢颠倒 6 次使血液与管内成分混匀,竖直立于 4℃冰箱内,并在 6 h 内进行血浆分离。低温(4℃),1 600×g 离心 10 min。离心完成后从离心机中取出样本,此时样本分为 3 层,下层为红细胞层,中间为白细胞和血小板,上层为所需的血浆。

吸取 2 ml 血浆置于 EP 管中。高速离心(6 000×g)10 min,提取上清液。

无创产前基因检测(noninvasive prenatal genetic testing,NIPT)文库构建,real-time PCR 扩增,高通量检测。

检查结果见表 12 - 1。

表 12 - 1　无创染色体检查结果

项目	检测值	正常值参考范围	检查结果
21 三体	18.120	<3	高风险
18 三体	1.632	<3	低风险
13 三体	0.531	<3	低风险

建议做羊水染色体检查。

(2)羊水染色体检查 Amniotic fluid examination:B 超监视下,用注射器经孕妇腹壁、子宫到羊膜腔抽取胎儿羊水 20～30 ml,将悬液均匀分配到无菌的培养瓶内,封口后置细胞培养箱培养;每隔几天用倒置显微镜观察生长情况,根据需要更换部分培养基;培养 15～20 d,当细胞铺满瓶壁时,收获细胞进行染色体分析(参加"人类染色体标本的制备"和"染色体 G 显带技术")。

检查结果:胎儿核型为 46,XY,+21

产前诊断:胎儿为 Down 综合征

Triple screen measurements in the maternal serum (AFP, 15 ng/ml; E$_3$, 17.7 mol/L; hCG, 4.62×10^3 IU/ml) and noninvasive prenatal genetic testing (NIPT) were performed and showed that the fetus had a high risk for chromosomal abnormalities. Therefore, amniotic fluid chromosome examination was performed (See "Human chromosome preparation" and "G banding").

Prenatal screenings (amniotic fluid chromosome examination):46, XY, +21

The prenatal diagnosis revealed that the fetus has Down syndrome.

二、遗传咨询与治疗　Genetic counseling and treatment

对李×的儿子和胎儿已作明确诊断,该疾病为染色体病(游离型),根据该病的性质、发病原理等特点,给予相应的遗传咨询。

(一)对策和措施　Prediction and suggestion

1. 告知与解释　Prediction

向李×解释诊断结果和产前诊断结果,告知该病的症状、原理、预后等情况,使其对 Down 综合征有充分的了解。

2. 建议和措施　Suggestion

因胎儿确诊为 Down 综合征,建议李×采用人工流产。但应由患者及其亲属自行做出决定,咨询医师不应替他们做出决定。

李×两次妊娠结果均为 Down 综合征,如再度妊娠,生育 Down 综合征的再发风险上升至 1‰～2‰(即 Down 综合征的发病率为 1/1 000～2/1 000)。建议如考虑再度怀孕的话,应再次作产前诊断。

(二) Down 综合征患儿治疗 Treatment

1. 生活技能和社会适应力的训练 Life skills and social adaptability training

Down 综合征患儿可经过训练学会读和写,以及基本的生活技能。也可试用谷氨酸、叶酸、维生素 B 等,对促进小儿智力发育,提高智商可能有一定的作用。

2. 其他临床症状的治疗 Other treatments

Down 综合征患儿常伴有先天性心脏病(如房间隔缺损与房室畸形),急性白血病的发病率也比较高,可进行相关的检查,如伴有类似临床症状的,进行相关治疗。先天性心脏病的可采取手术治疗。

(三) 随访 Follow-up

对咨询者进行随访,了解咨询的结果,特别是对李×是否选择人工流产、是否考虑再次受孕,进行随访,以便给予进一步的咨询。

The parents should discuss this option and reach a decision regarding the discontinuation of the pregnancy.

Down syndrome cannot be cured. However,early treatment can help many people with Down syndrome to live productive lives well into adulthood.

病例二 Case 2

姓名:金××　　性别:男　　出生日期:2006 年 11 月 20 日

民族:汉　　　　地址:上海市宝山区

就诊日期:2018 年 2 月

主诉:两年前起有视力模糊、减退,病程发展迅速。中心视力减退或丧失及视野缺损,但周围视力仍存在。

Name:Jin　　　Gander:Male　　Date of Birth:Nov 20th,2006

Address:Baoshan District,Shanghai

Date of hospital visit:February 2018

Chief complaint:Blurring and clouding of vision,and acute worsening of vision in both eyes. This condition mainly affected the central vision,and the patient still had preserved peripheral vision.

一、诊断 Diagnosis

(一) 临床诊断与家系分析 Clinical diagnosis and pedigree analysis

1. 检查 Examination

患者有中心视力严重减退,动态和静态的视野检查显示视野缺损、中心视力盲点,但周围视力仍存在。视盘充血、肿胀,表面毛细血管减少或丧失,视盘颜色浅淡,视网膜血管狭窄。诊断为视神经萎缩。

Ophthalmological diagnosis：Central vision acuity was severely reduced，visual field testing by kinetic or static perimetry showed centrocecal scotoma. Disk exhibited hyperemia and edema. Retinal vascular tortuosity and stenosis was obvious.

2. 病史与家族史采集　Medical history and family history review

病史见主诉：询问家族史得知患者家族中共有 8 人罹患视神经萎缩。

该病有明显家族聚集倾向，因此对患者家族作家系调查，分析其遗传方式。

The patient has a known family history of vision problems. An additional eight family members have the disease.

3. 家系调查与系谱分析　Pedigree analysis

对患者的家族进行家系调查，并绘制成系谱(图 12 - 1)。Ⅱ代中有两名患病，Ⅱ1 女性，72 岁，目前已失明。Ⅲ代中有 5 名患病，表现为不同程度的视力减退，均为Ⅱ1 的子女。

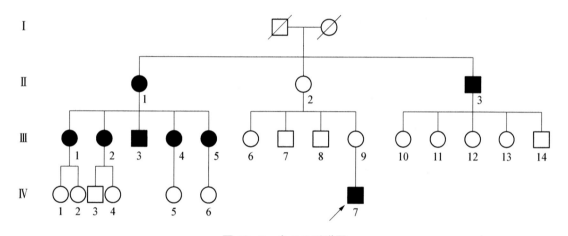

图 12 - 1　金××系谱图
Fig. 12 - 1　Pedigree of Jin's family

根据该系谱的特点：①男女均有发病；②三代均有患者出现；③女性患者将疾病传递给后代，而男性患者不能将疾病遗传给后代；④女性不发病，但其后代患病。可见致病基因来自于女性，男性生殖细胞对表型无作用，该家系的遗传方式不符合孟德尔遗传规律，而是呈现母系遗传；考虑其为线粒体遗传病，先证者的母亲和外祖母未出现症状，符合线粒体遗传多质性、异质性、阈值效应的特点。

根据系谱分析，此病的遗传方式为线粒体遗传。可能为线粒体遗传病 Leber 遗传性视神经病(Leber hereditary optic neuropathy，LHON)，为确诊，对先证者和家族其他患者进行基因诊断。

According to the pedigree analysis (Fig. 12 - 1), this disease exhibits mitochondrial inheritance and is possibly LHON. The diagnosis should be confirmed via the identification of a pathogenic mtDNA variant on molecular genetic testing of DNA extracted from a blood sample of the proband.

(二)基因诊断　Genetic diagnosis

诱发 LHON 的 mtDNA 突变均为点突变。如：G11778A、G14459A、G3460A、

T14484C 和 G15257A 等,都位于呼吸链酶复合物Ⅰ(ND1、ND2、ND4 和 ND5)和呼吸链酶复合物Ⅲ(Cyt C)的基因中。其中 G11778A 最为常见。

The mutations which cause LHON usually are point mutation like G11778A, G14459A, G3460A, T14484C, and G15257A. The mutant proteins are the part of the enzyme complexes in mitochondria such as ND1, ND4L, and ND6. The common mutation is G11778A.

1. PCR - RFLP 法检测线粒体基因 G11778A 突变　Detection of G11778A mutation of mitochondrial DNA by PCR-RFLP

(1) 抽取外周血,柠檬酸-葡萄糖(acid-citrate dextrose,ACD)抗凝剂抗凝。

(2) 抽提基因组 DNA(参见"真核细胞基因组 DNA 的提取")。

(3) PCR 扩增与限制性内切酶消化。

设计包含 mtDNA 11778 位的引物:

Primer1:5′- ATGGCAAGCCAACGCCACTT - 3′

Primer2:5′- CGTGGTTACTAGCACAGAGAGTTC - 3′

PCR 反应参数:94℃预变性 300 s,94℃变性 30 s,58℃退火 30 s,72℃延伸 30 s,共 30 个循环,末轮 72℃再延伸 300 s。

PCR 扩增产物 10 μl 加限制性内切酶 $SfaN$Ⅰ 4 U,37℃水浴消化 12 h。2% 琼脂糖凝胶电泳检测,凝胶成像分析仪成像拍照。

突变检测结果显示正常人 mtDNA11778 位点经 PCR 扩增后,可得到一条长 924 bp 的扩增片段,经 $SfaN$Ⅰ 酶切后可产生 797 bp 和 127 bp 两条片段。而 LHON 患者因 mtDNA 存在 G11778A 突变,酶切位点丢失,仍显示一条长 924 bp 的片段(图 12 - 2)。

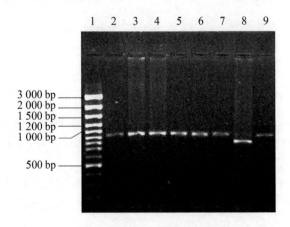

图 12 - 2　PCR 产物酶切后条带

Fig. 12 - 2　PCR products after digestion

1:标准分子量 Marker　2:mtDNA11778 PCR 扩增条带　3:无家族史患者酶切条带　4~9:家系成员酶切条带

检测证实患者 mtDNA11778 位点存在突变,可以确定是 Leber 视神经遗传病。也可以将 DNA 产物测序以进一步证实。

2. DNA 测序检测线粒体基因 G11778A 突变　Detection of G11778A mutation of

mitochondrial DNA by gene sequencing

先证者和 1 例正常人的 PCR 产物进行序列测定,并进行序列同源性分析。(http://PPwww. ncbi. nlm. nih. gov,人 *AY*714050 基因,mtDNA *ND*4 基因组 DNA)(图 12-3).

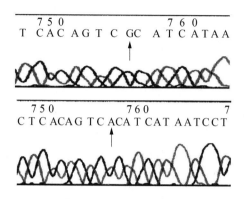

图 12-3　DNA 检测结果
Fig. 12-3　DNA sequencing result

对 LHON 家系中的先证者和 1 例正常人的 mtDNA 11778 PCR 产物进行测序,证实先证者确实存在 mtDNAG11778A 突变。

Gene diagnosis:A mtDNA G11778A mutation was detected by PCR-RFLP. The result was confirmed by gene sequencing.

二、遗传咨询与治疗　Genetic counseling and treatment

目前,Leber 视神经遗传病没有根治的方法,药物治疗和手术治疗只能为患者改善症状,但患者如已丧失视力,则没有良好的治疗措施。

(一)治疗　Treatment

1. 药物治疗　Medical treatement

药物中常用的包括神经营养药物如维生素 B$_1$、维生素 B$_{12}$、ATP 及辅酶 A 等,血管扩张药及活血化瘀药类如烟酸、地巴唑、维生素 E、维脑路通、复方丹参等。近年来,通过高压氧、体外反搏穴位注射东莨菪碱(654-2)等均已取得一定效果,中药及针刺治疗已证明有一定疗效,可继续应用发掘整理。尚应提及的是,禁止吸烟及饮烈性酒,增强机体体质。

2. 手术治疗　Surgical treatment

血管分流术、网膜血管再植术治疗,可使供应视神经及视网膜的眼动脉、视网膜中央动脉和睫状后短动脉的血流量增加,改善视神经及视网膜的缺血状态,丰富视神经及视网膜的营养,使患者的视力得到进一步提高和视野扩大。

对患者及家族成员已作明确诊断,该疾病为线粒体遗传病,根据该病的性质、发病原理等特点,给予相应的遗传咨询

(二)遗传咨询　Genetic counseling

1. 告知与解释　Prediction

将诊断结果向患者及家属解释,告知该病的症状、原理、预后等情况,使其对本病有充分了解。

2. 再发风险估计　Recurrence risk estimation

Leber 视神经遗传病一般成年期发病,平均年龄为 27 岁,但最早可在 6 岁,最晚可在 60 岁发病。因此,Ⅳ的 1～6 仍存在再发风险。Ⅱ2 为致病突变的携带者,其子女Ⅲ6～9 具有再发风险,但是线粒体病有遗传异质性、多质性和不均等有丝分裂的特点,所以Ⅲ6～9 也可能不发病,同时因Ⅲ6～9 的年龄都已超过 35 岁,所以发病风险进一步降低。但其后代仍存在再发风险。Ⅱ3 为男性患者,线粒体病呈母系遗传,所以其后代不会罹患此病。

3. 建议和措施　Suggestion

根据系谱分析和本病的遗传规律,给予该家族成员相应的建议,对具有再发风险的家族成员可及早进行基因诊断,做到早诊断、早治疗。

4. 随访　Follow-up

对患者家族进行随访,了解发病情况和就诊情况,提供必要的进一步咨询。

The treatment of LHON includes general therapies for mitochondrial disorders and anti-apoptotic agents (antioxidant, a vitamin E derivative).

Genetic counseling: The mother of the proband would transmit a considerable amount of mutant mtDNA to the offspring if she planned to have a new baby. Although some of the proband's maternal relatives are unaffected by the disease, they still might carry the mutant mtDNA, which represents a theoretical risk of transmitting the disease to their offspring.

病例三　Case 3

姓名:朱××　　性别:女　　出生日期:1998 年 1 月 13 日

民族:汉　　　　地址:上海市闸北区

就诊日期:2018 年 3 月

主诉:家族中有 4 人已患有某种神经系统疾病,症状表现为不由自主地舞蹈样动作,病程逐渐加重,其中一人为朱××的外祖母(65 岁),朱××的母亲目前未见异常,朱××希望知道自己是否会发病。

Name: Zhu　　Gander: Female　　Date of Birth: Jan 13th, 1998

Address: Zhabei District, Shanghai

Date of hospital visit: March 2018

Chief complaint: Miss Zhu had a known family history of a type of neurological disorder, and four family members had the disease, including her grandmother (who is 65 years old). The symptoms were unsteady gait and involuntary movements. Zhu's mother has not exhibited symptoms. Miss Zhu consulted us regarding the possibility of her having the disease.

一、诊断　Diagnosis

(一)家系分析　Pedigree analysis

1. 家族史采集　Family history review

病史见主诉；询问家族史得知患者家族中共有 4 人罹患该病。

该病有明显家族聚集倾向，因此对患者家族进行家系调查，分析其遗传方式。

2. 家系调查与系谱分析 Pedigree analysis

对患者的家族进行家系调查，并绘制成系谱（图 12-4）。

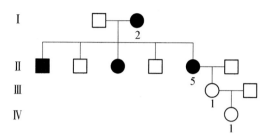

图 12-4 朱×× 系谱图
Fig. 12-4 Pedigree of zhu's family

根据该系谱的特点：①男女皆有发病；②系谱中连续传递；③患者的双亲中有一方为患者；估计该病为常染色体显性遗传。

根据系谱该病遗传方式为常染色体显性遗传，结合临床表现，怀疑为亨廷顿病（Huntington disease，HD），即 Huntington 病，对家族中的患者作基因诊断以确诊。

The pedigree shows the disease is autosomal dominant. The clinical characteristic and the inheritance mode suggest it is Huntington disease.

（二）基因诊断 Genetic diagnosis

Huntington 病是常染色体显性遗传病，为 4 号染色体短臂 4p16.3 的 *HTT* 基因突变所致，基因产物为 CAG 三核苷酸重复扩增产生 Huntington 蛋白，正常人为 19～38 个 CAG 重复序列，HD 为 40 个以上。本病的遗传特点包括早现现象：连续后代中有发病年龄提前倾向；父系遗传的早发倾向更明显。

Mutations in the *HTT* gene cause Huntington disease. The *HTT* mutation that causes Huntington disease is a CAG trinucleotide repeat that is called a dynamic mutation. Normally, the CAG segment is repeated 19 to 38 times within the gene. In patients with Huntington disease, the CAG segment is repeated more than 40 times. The diseases that are caused by CAG trinucleotide repeat expansion exhibit a phenomenon termed anticipation. As the mutant gene is passed from one generation to the next, the size of the trinucleotide repeat will increase, which means an earlier onset of the signs and symptoms of the disease.

1. 提取外周血 DNA Blood DNA extraction

该家系中 I 2 已故，II 2 因故未能采集血样，II 5、III 1、IV 1 抽取外周血，抽提基因组 DNA。

2. PCR 扩增 CAG 片段 Amplification of CAG repeat region by PCR

设计引物：

上游引物(HD1)5′ATGAAG2GCCTTCGAGTCCCTCAAGTCCTTC 3′

下游引物(HD3)5′GGCGGTGGCGGCTGTTGCTGCTGCTGCTGC 3′

PCR 反应参数:94℃预变性 1 min,94℃变性 30 s,58℃退火 30 s,72℃延伸 2 min,共 30 个循环,末轮 72℃再延伸 10 min。

3. 测定 CAG 重复数 Determination of CAG repeats

取 20 μl PCR 产物进行 6%的变性聚丙烯酰胺凝胶电泳(常温,400 V,3 h)。电泳后银染凝胶,CAG 重复数可在银染后通过与 DNA 分子标记物(Marker),进行比较推算(当 PCR 产物长度为 104 bp 时,重复数为 19)。

3 名患者(Ⅱ5,Ⅲ1,Ⅳ1)都各有一个等位基因的 CAG 重复数超过了 40,分别为 57、49 和 63。

基因诊断证实该家系中的患者患有 Huntington 病,根据其遗传特征对朱××进行基因分析和遗传咨询。

Extract DNA from the Peripheral blood, PCR amplification of CAG fragments. The results confirmed that the family of the proband suffered from Huntington disease.

二、遗传咨询与治疗 Genetic counseling and treatment

(一)患者治疗 Treatment

本病目前尚无法治愈。运动障碍和舞蹈症可对纹状体输出神经元多巴胺能抑制药物有反应,包括:①多巴胺 D_2-受体阻断剂:氟哌啶醇、氯丙嗪、泰必利等;②耗竭神经末梢多巴胺的药物:利血平、丁苯那嗪等;③选择性 5-羟色胺再摄取抑制剂可能减轻病情进展;增强 γ-氨基丁酸(GABA)能和胆碱能神经传递药物通常无效。

(二)遗传咨询 Genetic counseling

随访和扩大咨询。对患者家族其他成员可进行随访,对再发风险高的个体进行基因诊断,以做到早诊断早治疗。

Although there is no cure for HD, there are treatments available to reduce the severity of some of its symptoms. The drugs used to manage HD include ① dopamine D_2-receptor blockers: haloperidol, chlorpromazine; ② Tetrabenazine, its anti-chorea effect is attributed to a reversible depletion of monoamines, such as dopamine, serotonin, norepinephrine, and histamine, from nerve terminals; ③ Selective serotonin reuptake inhibitors.

（刘 雯）

第十三章　遗传病的生物信息分析实验

Bioinformatics methods for analysis of genetic diseases

在医学遗传学中，生物信息学的关键是认识基因的确切位置和各序列的功能，了解其调控机制，从而描述人类疾病的内在规律。使用生物信息学阐释人类遗传疾病，已经成为现代遗传疾病诊断中不可或缺的方法。本章将简要介绍测序及分析的原理、生物信息学的常用数据库、生物信息学分析的基本概念及方法，并以病例的形式对人类遗传病开展生物信息分析实验。

In medical genetics, the key role of bioinformatics is the identification of the exact location of genes and the functions of each sequence, therefore, so that geneticists can understand the regulatory mechanisms of human diseases. The use of bioinformatics to interpret human genetic diseases has become an indispensable method in the diagnosis of modern genetic diseases. In this chapter, we will briefly introduce the principles of sequencing and analysis, the common database of bioinformatics, the basic concepts and methods of bioinformatics analysis, and a case analysis using bioinformatics.

第一节 ◎ 后基因组计划时代的遗传学分析
Genetic analysis in the post-genome era

一、概述　Overview

2003 年，人类基因组计划宣告基本完成。十年后，有记者问，在医药和人类健康方面人们是否从该计划获益良多？公共计划的领导者 Francis Collins 和私营计划的领导者 Craig Venter 均回答"不是很多"[Nature editorial staff. （2010）The human genome at ten. Nature，464：649 - 650.]。在后基因组时代，遗传学家理解了基因组的"解剖结构"，需要进一步了解基因的功能，才能使用生物信息学阐释人类疾病。后基因组计划时代，人类基因组研究已进入了信息提取和数据分析的全新阶段。

In 2003, the Human Genome Project (HGP) was declared to be completed. In the post-HGP era, geneticists further want to understand the function of genes. Human genome research has entered a new phase of information extraction and data analysis.

二、测序技术　Sequencing

弗雷德·桑格尔(Fred Sanger)于 1977 年发表了一代测序方法,并第二次获得诺贝尔化学奖。该法昂贵费时,测序第一个人类基因组的花费将近 27 亿美金。2000 年后诞生的第二代测序技术,主要特点是多分子测序、需扩增、序列读长短。该技术将人类基因组测序的成本逐渐降至 1 000 美金,使得基因组测序的广泛应用成为可能。Illumina 公司在 2007 年的基因组分析仪是二代测序的代表仪器。第三代测序技术如 Pacific Biosciences 公司的单分子实时测序 Single Molecule Real-Time(SMRT)等,其特点是单分子测序、依赖 DNA 聚合酶的活性。目前,在人类基因组测序中得到广泛应用的是第二代测序方法。

Fred Sanger published the first generation of sequencing methods in 1977 and won the Nobel Prize in Chemistry for the second time. In 2000, the second generation of sequencing technologies was developed. This technology has gradually reduced the cost of sequencing human genomes to 1 000 USD. Illumina's Genomic Analyzer is the representative instrument of second-generation sequencing. Third-generation sequencing technologies, such as Pacific Biosciences' single-molecule real-time sequencing (SMRT), are characterized by single-molecule sequencing.

在整个人类基因组中,蛋白质编码区域仅占 1%,约 30 Mb。被分为 180 000 个外显子区。孟德尔疾病是由一对等位基因控制的疾病或病理性状,人体中只要单个基因发生突变就足以发病的一类遗传性疾病。目前,绝大多数已知导致孟德尔疾病的突变位于外显子编码区内。因此,为方便高效、价格低廉地进行检测,人们设计了富集方法,捕获所有蛋白质编码外显子的序列。其原理是:构建生物素化的寡核苷酸探针,从生成的文库中杂交捕获目标序列。之后与带有链霉抗生物素的磁珠结合,并清洗掉未结合的片段。富集得到的片段通过常用的衔接序列,经 PCR 扩增,制备文库。从而进行全外显子测序。这一方法一般捕获所有外显子区及其侧翼序列,也可包括 miRNA 和其他感兴趣的序列。目前常用的有 Agilent 公司及艾吉泰康公司的捕获试剂盒。

The protein-coding region accounts for only 1% (30 Mb, 180 000 exonic regions) of the entire human genome. An enrichment method was designed to capture the sequence of all protein-encoding exons. This method typically captures all exon regions and their flanking sequences, and may also include miRNAs and other sequences of interest. At present, Agilent's and iGeneTech's capture kits are commonly used.

目前最常用的二代测序 Illumina 技术,主要包括 3 个步骤,即:文库制备、流动室制备和合成测序。

Currently, the most commonly used second-generation sequencing, the Illumina technology, includes three main steps: library preparation, flow-cell preparation and sequencing by synthesis.

(一)文库制备　Library preparation

文库制备是创建一个包含随机 DNA 片段的库,用于测序。这是二代测序与桑格尔测序的重要区别。这需要对某些 DNA 片段进行扩增。扩增可通过特异性引物 PCR 或使用分子克隆引入通用引物结合序列。由于长片段的放大效率较低,难以在流动室表面集群,一般要求待测 DNA 片段小于 800 个核苷酸(nt)。

Library preparation requires the amplification of certain DNA fragments. Amplification can be introduced into universal primer-binding sequences by specific primer PCR or using molecular cloning.

建库一般再分为 4 个步骤(图 13 - 1):

Library preparation includes (Fig. 13 - 1):

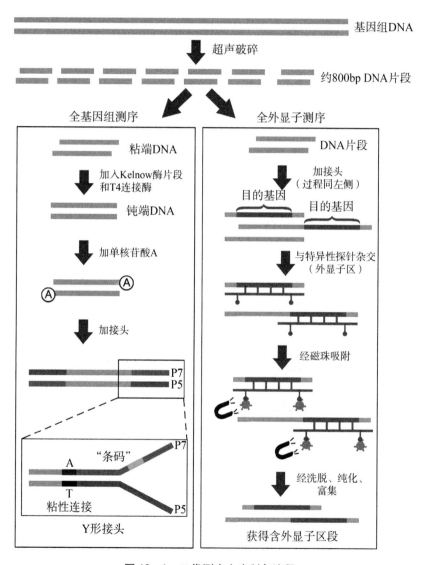

图 13 - 1 二代测序文库制备流程

Fig. 13 - 1 Next-generation sequencing library preparation

1. DNA 片段化 Fragmentation

超声处理产生微小气泡,产生剪切力,使 DNA 分裂成大小均匀的片段。

2. 断端修复并添加单个腺嘌呤(A)尾 End repair and addition of an A overhang

片段化后,DNA 片段末端可以具有 5'或 3'突出端,这将阻止后续的酶促步骤。使用 T4 DNA 聚合酶和来自大肠杆菌 DNA 聚合酶 I 的 Klenow 区段,可以达到 DNA 片段的"抛光"。随后将单个腺嘌呤(A)核苷酸添加到钝的 3'末端,防止 DNA 片段相互连接。这一步骤通过添加 dATP 和 Klenow 外切酶活性缺失片段(Klenow exo- Fragment)达成。

3. 添加适配片段 Adapter ligation

适配片段是化学合成的短链双链 DNA,与随机 DNA 片段连接,在随机片段两端提供恒定序列。适配片段是多用途的,两个适配片段设计为 Y 形,可结合在库片段的任意一端,允许特异性的 PCR 富集。适配片段含有与流动室的结合区,还可以引入索引或者条码(barcode)。

4. 选择连接的 DNA Select ligation of DNA

适配片段与末端修复的加 A 尾 DNA 按 10∶1 混合,通过 T4 DNA 连接酶连接。经纯化去除未连接的适配片段二聚体。随后通过 PCR 有选择地富集两端均带有适配片段的 DNA。PCR 后需要验证库中 DNA 的量和纯度。带有不同条码的 DNA 片段可以合并统计。

(二) **流动室制备 Flow-cell preparation**

流动室本质上是一个玻璃片,带有一个或多个通道。每个通道均涂有与适配片段互补的寡核苷酸链(既有与 5'端互补也有与 3'端互补)。PCR 产物经过氢氧化钠处理变性后,单链 DNA 分子与寡核苷酸链互补锚定。然后,扩增混合物(缓冲液、dNTPs、DNA 聚合酶)流入,产生双链分子。其中只有一条链是共价连接在玻片上的。洗脱掉非共价连接的链后,通过桥式扩增获得多个"菌落"样、约 1 000 个产物、两端均在玻片上的 DNA 桥。

测序反应只能在一个方向上执行。因此,反向链被切割并丢弃,留下具有前向链的簇。通过末端转移酶将脱氧核苷酸加到 3'羟基末端阻断,防止干扰后续的测序反应(图 13 - 2)。

The flow-cell tool is essentially a piece of glass coated with an oligonucleotide strand complementary to the adaptor fragment. After bridge amplification, a plurality of "colony"-like DNA bridges of about 1 000 products with both ends on the slide are obtained for further sequencing steps.

(三) **合成测序 Sequencing by synthesis**

合成测序(sequencing by synthesis,SBS)需要先添加测序引物,此引物对应于适配序列的一个区域。使用带有特定荧光标记的 dNTP - 3'- OH 进行单碱基测序。其中 3'- OH 基团是可逆性的化学终止基团。激光激发后,记录特定荧光。单碱基测序完成后解除阻断,可以进行下一个 dNTP - 3'- OH 结合。

Sequencing by synthesis (SBS) requires the addition of sequencing primers corresponding to a region of the adaptor sequence. Single-base sequencing is performed using fluorescent labeled dNTPs with a 3'- OH blocking group. Specific fluorescence is recorded upon laser excitation. After the single-base sequencing is completed,the blocking group is released and the next cycle begins.

理论上,完美的测序周期应该产生强烈的单碱基信号而没有其他 3 个碱基的信号。然而真实情况并非如此,需通过特定的算法滤除杂信号。对于加了条码的适配片段,测序时需使

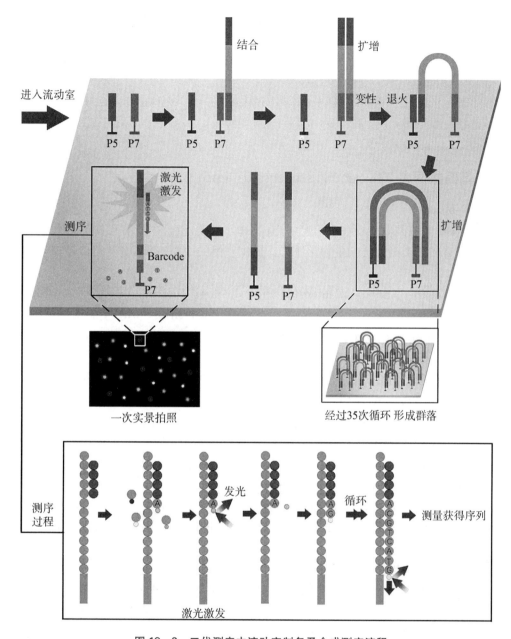

图 13 - 2 二代测序中流动室制备及合成测序流程

Fig. 13 - 2 Flow-cell preparation and sequencing by synthesis in next-generation sequencing

用特定的测序引物对条码进行测序。

第二节 ◉ 生物信息分析相关数据库
Bioinformatics-related database

目前,世界上数以百计的生物信息数据库,按特定目标收集生物学实验数据,并提供相关服务。大多数可免费访问。对医学遗传学较重要的著名数据库包括：一级数据库（原始数据）：核酸数据：Genbank；蛋白质数据：UniProt、PDB 等；二级数据库（针对特定目标对实验数据整理得到）：功能数据库：京都基因和基因组百科全书（KEGG）；遗传病数据库：OMIM；变异与表型数据库：ClinVar、HGMD 等。

There are hundreds of bioinformatics databases in the world. These databases collect biological experimental data and provide related services according to specific goals. Most of them are free of access.

一、基因数据库　Nucleotide sequence database

（一）Genbank

Genbank 由美国国立生物技术信息中心（NCBI）建立，包含了所有已知的核酸序列和蛋白质序列，具有相关文献链接和生物学注释。提供广泛的数据查询、序列相似性搜索以及其他分析服务。

Founded by the National Center for Biotechnology Information（NCBI），GenBank contains all known nucleic acid sequences and protein sequences，with associated literature links and biological annotations. It provides extensive data query，sequence similarity search，and other analytical services.

Genbank 库里的数据按来源于约 55 000 个物种，其中 56% 是人类的基因组序列。每条 Genbank 数据记录包含了对序列的简要描述，它的科学命名，物种分类名称，参考文献，序列特征表，以及序列本身。序列特征表里包含对序列生物学特征注释，如：编码区、转录单元、重复区域、突变位点或修饰位点等。

Each GenBank data record contains a brief description of the sequence，including the scientific nomenclature，the species classification name，the reference，the sequence characteristics table，and the sequence itself. It also contains annotations of sequence biological features，such as coding regions，transcription units，repeated regions，mutation sites，or modification sites.

1. Genbank 数据检索

NCBI 的数据库检索查询系统是 Entrez。Entrez 是基于 Web 界面的综合生物信息数据库检索系统。利用 Entrez 系统，用户不仅可以方便地检索 Genbank 的核酸数据，还可以交叉检索来自 Genbank 和其他数据库的蛋白质序列数据、基因组图谱数据、来自分子模型数据库（MMDB）的蛋白质三维结构数据、种群序列数据集、以及由 PubMed 获得 Medline 的文献数据。详细的 Entrez 使用说明可以在该主页上获得。

2. 向 Genbank 提交序列数据

测序工作者可把新序列添加到 Genbank 数据库。使用 BankIt 应用可提交序列信息及序列相关信息。相关网址：https://www.ncbi.nlm.nih.gov/genbank/。

二、蛋白质数据库 Protein database

（一）UniProt

UniProt 是经过注释的蛋白质序列数据库，由欧洲生物信息学研究所（EBI）、瑞士生物信息学研究所（SIB）、蛋白质信息资源（PIR）联合建立。整合了 Swiss-Prot 等多个蛋白质资源数据库。每个条目包含蛋白质序列、文献信息、分类学信息、注释等，注释中包括蛋白质的功能、特殊位点和区域、二级结构、四级结构与其他序列的相似性、序列残缺与疾病的关系、序列变异体和冲突等信息。并与核酸序列库、蛋白质序列库和蛋白质结构库等做了交叉引用。序列提交可以在其 Web 页面上完成。相关网址：https://www. uniprot. org。

UniProt is an annotated database of protein sequences created by the European Institute of Bioinformatics (EBI), the Swiss Institute of Bioinformatics (SIB), and the Protein Information Resources (PIR). Each entry contains protein sequences, literature information, taxonomic information, annotations, etc. The annotations include protein function, specific sites and regions, secondary structure, related disease information, etc.

（二）PDB

蛋白质数据库（protein database，PDB）是生物大分子结构数据库，由结构生物信息学研究合作组织（RCSB）维护。PDB 收集的数据来源于 X 线晶体衍射和核磁共振（nuclear magnetic resonance，NMR）的数据，经过整理和确认后存档而成。使用 Rasmol 等软件可以在计算机上按 PDB 文件显示生物大分子的三维结构。相关网址：http://www. rcsb. org。

The Protein Database (PDB) is a database of biological macromolecular structures maintained by the Association of Structural Bioinformatics Research (RCSB). The data collected by PDB was derived from X-ray crystal diffraction and nuclear magnetic resonance (NMR) data, which were archived after confirmation.

三、功能数据库 Functional database

（一）KEGG

京都基因和基因组百科全书（KEGG）是系统分析基因功能，联系基因组信息和功能信息的知识库。基因组信息存储在 GENES 数据库里，包括完整和部分测序的基因组序列；更高级的功能信息存储在 PATHWAY 数据库里，包括图解的细胞生化过程如代谢、膜转运、信号传递、细胞周期，还包括同系保守的子通路等信息。KEGG 提供图形工具来访问基因组图谱，比较基因组图谱和操作表达图谱，还可进行序列比较、图形比较和通路计算。相关网址：http://www. genome. ad. jp/kegg/。

The Kyoto Encyclopedia of Genes and Genomes (KEGG) is a knowledge base that systematically analyzes gene function and links genomic information to functional information. Genomic information is stored in the GENES database, while functional information is stored in the PATHWAY database, including graphical cellular biochemical processes such as metabolism, membrane transport, signaling, cell cycle, and homologous conservation.

(二) OMIM

人类孟德尔遗传学(OMIM)是人类基因和遗传表型的全面权威的数据库,包含所有已知孟德尔病症和超过 15 000 个基因的信息。OMIM 专注于表型和基因型之间的关系,由约翰霍普金斯医学院维护。OMIM 为每个条目提供唯一的六位数标识符,是遗传疾病的稳定标识。相关网址:https://www.omim.org/。

The Online Mendelian Inheritance in Man (OMIM) is a comprehensive, authoritative database of human genetic and phenotypic information. It contains information on all known Mendelian disorders and more than 15 000 genes. OMIM provides a unique six-digit identifier for each entry. The identifier is a stable marker for genetic diseases.

(三) ClinVar

ClinVar 是人类变异和表型关系的数据库,提供人类变异的报告,及其表型支持证据。变异识别的精准性和其临床意义的可信度在很大程度上取决于支持证据,ClinVar 汇总相关信息,反映对相关变异的认识。

ClinVar 包含患者样本中发现的变异、临床意义、提交者信息及其他支持数据。等位基因与参考序列比对后,根据 HGVS 标准列出。提交报告有多种形式,包括变异提交、案例提交、实验证据提交等。ClinVar 包括了 OMIM、dbSNP、和其他数据源。相关网址:https://www.ncbi.nlm.nih.gov/clinvar/。

ClinVar is a database of human variability and phenotypic relationships, providing reports of human variation and evidence of phenotypic support. It aggregates relevant information to reflect the understanding of the relevant variation. ClinVar contains mutations, clinical significance, submitter information, and other supporting data found in patient samples. The variations are listed according to the HGVS standard.

(四) HGMD

人类基因突变数据库(The Human Gene Mutation Database,HGMD)创建于 1996 年,全面收集与人类遗传疾病相关的基因突变。此数据库系统地收录文献中的所有致病突变和与疾病相关的功能多态性,包括单碱基置换(比如,编码序列中的错义突变、无义突变、以及调控和剪切区域中的点突变)、微缺失(micro-deletions)和微插入(micro-insertions)、缺失/插入(indels)、重复序列扩增以及大的基因损伤(缺失、插入和倍增)和更复杂的基因重组等。相较于 ClinVar,HGMD 变异位点覆盖更为全面,但其近年更新的数据需要付费获得。相关网址:http://www.hgmd.cf.ac.uk/ac/index.php/。

Created in 1996, the Human Gene Mutation Database (HGMD) comprehensively collects genetic mutations associated with human genetic diseases. This database systematically contains all pathogenic mutations and disease-related functional polymorphisms available in the literature, including single-base-pair substitutions in coding (e. g., missense and nonsense), regulatory and splicing-relevant regions of human nuclear genes, micro-deletions and micro-insertions, indels, repeat expansions, as well as gross gene lesions (deletions, insertions, and duplications) and complex gene rearrangements. Compared with ClinVar, the HGMD comprehensively covers more genetic mutations. However，access to its updated data in recent years requires payment.

第三节 ◉ 生物信息分析相关数据格式、软件和概念
Bioinformatics-related data formats and software

生物信息学分析在实践中是十分复杂的。需要考虑到硬件、测序系统、测序质量等多项参数。进行分析之前需要对原始数据去重、去除低质量测序结果进行质控。分析时需要调节多种参数，才能做到良好的变异识别。我们在这一节介绍生物信息分析的常见概念。

Bioinformatics analysis is complicated in practice. Many parameters，such as hardware，sequencing system，and sequencing quality，need to be considered. Prior to analysis，the raw data need to be deduplicated，low-quality sequencing results need to be removed，and quality control must be performed. During the analysis，a variety of parameters require adjustment to achieve good variant calling.

一、BCL 文件 BCL file

Illumina 测序仪执行图像分析和碱基识别，输出 ∗. bcl 文件。Illumina 测序仪的仪器控制软件执行图像分析，定位序列簇，并输出测序强度、XY 定位、噪声估算等信息。碱基识别由仪器执行。在生物信息学操作中，需要使用 bcl2fastq2 软件将其转换为可操作的 ∗. fastq. gz 文件，并将复合样本按条码分离为不同的 ∗. fastq. gz 文件。

软 件 下 载 地 址：https://support. illumina. com/downloads/bcl2fastq-conversion-software-v2-20. html

The Illumina sequencer performs image analysis and base identification and outputs ∗. bcl files. The Bcl2fastq2 software is required to convert ∗. bcl files into an operational ∗. fastq. gz file.

二、FASTQ 文件 FASTQ file

FASTQ 是测序数据文件格式，包含了序列信息和每个碱基的质量得分。其名称源自 FASTA 文件格式，这是最初表示 DNA 和氨基酸序列的格式。这一格式在生物信息学中十分通用。第一行具有">"符号，后有名称和序列号。第二行起具有序列信息。FASTQ 格式是 FASTA 格式的扩展，额外储存了每个碱基的质量得分。在生物信息学操作中，可能需要先使用 FastQC 软件进行数据质量控制。使用 Trimmomatic 软件去除适配序列的污染等。

软件下载地址：

https://www. bioinformatics. babraham. ac. uk/projects/fastqc/

http://www. usadellab. org/cms/? page＝trimmomatic

FASTQ is a sequencing data file format that contains sequence information and a quality score for each base. It is an extension of the FASTA format that additionally stores the quality score. The FastQC software can be used for data quality control. The Trimmomatic software is used to remove contaminations.

三、参考基因组　Reference genome

遗传学生物信息分析的目的是对测序的个体基因组与参考基因组进行比对,确定其差异。由于具有参考基因组,比对算法无须从头组合拼接各 DNA 片段,比对过程快速而准确。人类参考基因组是最高质量的动物基因组之一,现已达到 38 版(GRCh38),不过仍有部分研究者使用 hg19 版本。参考基因组文件不仅含有主要染色体的序列,还有以下序列数据。①Random contigs:已知起源于特定染色体,但未准确定位的序列(如 chr9_KI270720v1_random)。②ChrUn:已知来源于人类但未定位到特定染色体的序列。③EBV:Epstein-Barr 病毒序列,如疱疹病毒 4 型,约 98% 的成年人已经接触过该病毒,在人类基因组中非常常见。④HLA:人白细胞抗原(HLA)序列,编码主要组织相容性复合物(MHC),在群体中变化很大。⑤Decoy sequences:诱饵序列。若样本包含了不在参考基因组中的片段,比对过程会花费大量时间寻找匹配。若该段与一个诱饵序列匹配,则可以被分配至此,防止无用的比对,避免错误。⑥Alternative contigs:替代序列,针对复杂结构变异。

软件下载地址:

ftp://hgdownload. soe. ucsc. edu/goldenPath/hg19

ftp://hgdownload. soe. ucsc. edu/goldenPath/hg38

https://www. ncbi. nlm. nih. gov/grc/human

The purpose of variant calling is to compare the sequenced individual genome with the reference genome to determine the difference. The Human Reference Genome is one of the highest quality animal genomes and has now reached version 38(GRCH38).

四、SAM/BAM 文件　SAM/BAM file

序列比对/映射(Sequence Alignment/Map (SAM))格式是存储二代测序的比对结果的通用格式。BAM(Binary Alignment/Map)格式是其二进制版本。可以使用 SAMtools、Picard 等软件对其进行操作。

软件下载地址:

http://samtools. sourceforge. net/

https://broadinstitute. github. io/picard/

The Sequence Alignment/Map (SAM) format is a common format for storing alignment results for second-generation sequencing. The Binary Alignment/Map (BAM) format is a compressed version of SAM files. It can be operated using software such as SAMtools or Picard.

五、基因组分析工具包　Genome analysis toolkit

基因组分析工具包(genome analysis toolkit,GATK)是使用最广泛的变异识别工具之一,是一个大型软件包,在变异识别之前也可以提高比对质量,校正碱基质量。是常见的比对后分析工具。在使用 GATK 之前可能需要使用 Picard 软件对 BAM 数据进行前处理。GATK 功能强大且复杂,本书仅作简介。GATK 的命令结构基本相同,计算 BAM 文件的序列读数命令如下：

```
java -jar GenomeAnalysisTK. jar \
-T CountReads \
-R example_reference. fasta \
-I example_reads. bam
```

其中-jar 函数调用 GATK 引擎,-T 函数运行特定工具,-R 函数调用参考基因组,-I 函数指定输入文件。

软件下载地址：

https://software. broadinstitute. org/gatk/

The genome analysis toolkit (GATK) is a large software package that is widely used for variant calling. BAM data may need to be pre-processed using the Picard software before input into GATK. The code for variant calling from a BAM file is as follows：

```
Java -jar GenomeAnalysisTK. jar \
-T CountReads \
-R example_reference. fasta \
-I example_reads. bam
```

The -jar function calls the GATK engine，the -T function runs a specific tool，the -R function calls the reference genome，and the -I function specifies the input file.

六、测序深度和捕获效率　Sequencing depth and capture efficiency

测序深度是判断全基因组/全外显子组测序质量的关键参数。对于参考基因组中某个给定碱基,深度即包含该碱基的序列数量。深度越深,对基因型的判定就越可信。在遗传学分析中,全基因组/全外显子组测序的目的是发现变异,需要较强的深度。若深度达到 100 倍,我们发现 48 个变异读数和 52 个非变异读数,则可判定其是杂合子。捕获效率体现了外显子组富集的效果,即靶向的区域与非靶向的区域相比,富集了多少倍。一般要求在 25 倍以上。

Sequencing depth and coverage are two key parameters for determining the quality of WES/WGS sequencing. For a given base in the reference genome, the depth means the number of sequences that containing a certain base. The deeper the depth，the more confident the genotyping. Capture efficiency reflects the effect of exome enrichment. A coverage of more than 25 times is generally required for WES.

七、变异识别

变异识别是指与参考基因组对照,识别出变异的过程。现有软件可对小变异(小于 50 nt)进行识别,也可对更大的结构变体进行识别。GATK 中的 HaplotypeCaller 模块常用于变异识别,适合单样本或多样本分析。从比对好的 BAM 进行变异识别的命令如下：

```
java -jar GenomeAnalysisTK. jar \
-T HaplotypeCaller \
```

-R hs38DH. fa \
-I NIST7035_indelrealigner. bam \
--genotyping_mode DISCOVERY \
-stand_call_conf 30 \
-o raw_variants. vcf

其中-jar 函数调用 GATK 引擎,-T 函数运行 HaplotypeCaller,-R 函数调用参考基因组 hs38DH. fa,-I 函数指定输入文件 NIST7035_indelrealigner. bam,--genotyping_mode(长形式函数)定义进行基因型分析的模式,-stand_call_conf 设定识别阈值,-o 指定输出文件为 raw_variants. vcf。

HaplotypeCaller 模块首先确定有变化的基因组,定义为活跃区域。随后识别特定的单倍型。最后计算给定数据的单倍型概率,分配最可能的基因型。

Variant call refers to the process of identifying differences compared with a reference genome. GATK can identify small variations (less than 50 nt) and larger structural variants. The HaplotypeCaller module in GATK is often used for variant calling.

八、变异识别格式 Variant call format

变异识别软件识别出的序列变体存储在 *. vcf 文件中。变异识别格式(variant call format,VCF)文件有两个主要部分,元信息部分和数据部分,由列标题行分隔。VCF 文件可以代表基因型信息,与 FASTQ 文件、SAM/BAM 文件构成了全基因组/全外显子组测序数据的分析三要素。

The sequence variants called by variant caller software are stored in the *. vcf file. AVCF file has two main parts, a meta-information part and a data part. The VCF file, the FASTQ file, and the SAM/BAM file constitute the three elements of the analysis of WES/WGS data.

九、变异注释 Variation annotation

要得到较好的数据,必须对变异命名法进行标准化。如今变异的注释基本采用人类基因组变异学会(Human Genome Variation Society,HGVS)的标准。遗传学研究中侧重于序列变异的鉴定,并将其与疾病相关联。其中关键的步骤是注释。例如,chr15:g. 48463207T>C 表示 15 号染色体上基因组 48 463 207 位点 T 变为 C。或 NM 000138. 4(FBN1):c. 5099A>G 表示 NM 000138. 4 *FBN1* 基因的 cDNA5099 位点 A 变为 G。而 p. (Y1700C)则表示蛋白中 1 700 位氨基酸由酪氨酸变为半胱氨酸。HGVS 网站提供了变异命名标准(http://varnomen. hgvs. org)。

The variant nomenclature must be standardized. Annotations generally use the standards of the Human Genome Variation Society (HGVS). For example, chr15:g. 48463207T > C indicates that, on chromosome 15, the genomic 48463207 site T becomes C.

十、变异和结构变体　Variation and structural variants

典型的人类基因组与人类参考基因组比较分析,具有超过 400 万个单核苷酸变异(SNVs)以及数千种结构变体(structural variation,SVs)。由于二代测序主要是一些短序列测序,要精准而全面地检测 SVs 十分困难。大约 50％的人类基因组由重复序列组成,这些重复序列易于进行基因组重排。

A typical human genome contains more than 4 million single-nucleotide variants (SNVs) and thousands of structural variants (SVs). Because of the short sequencing fragments, it is difficult to detect SVs accurately.

十一、变异致病性预测　Variant pathogenicity prediction

外显子组通常含有数以万计的 DNA 变体,其中有数千种错义突变、数百种无义突变、剪切位点突变和功能丢失突变。通常情况下,其中有数百种突变是罕见或仅见的。判断外显子突变的致病可能性非常困难。ClinVar 是医学相关突变的数据集。在记录的数十万突变中,约 30％为意义不明,18％为可能有害,我们仅能认定其中不到一半的突变。而这些与实际测序中得到的突变比起来也仅是一小部分。所以,我们需要对突变进行预测。通过评估蛋白质编码基因突变,对氨基酸的疏水性、电荷、序列和蛋白结构等进行预测。这一过程可以通过 SIFT、Polyphen、MutationTaster 等软件进行。需要注意的是,针对单独的蛋白质或基因产物进行的预测不足以鉴定疾病因果。若不考虑其假阳性可能会导致严重的后果。用户必须考虑临床证据做出最终诊断。

Typical exomes usually contain tens of thousands of DNA variants, including thousands of missense mutations, hundreds of nonsense mutations, cleavage site mutations, and loss of function mutations. ClinVar is a data set of medically relevant mutations. Variant pathogenicity prediction can be performed using the MutationTaster and other software.

十二、变体优先级　Variant priority

二代测序对于精准医疗变得越来越重要,但基于 NGS 对罕见遗传病的诊断并不是万能的。实际上,在大样本中,使用这一方法,其检出率仅达到 1/4。在分析中可能需要对突变进行优先级排序,确定其与特定疾病的相关性。这需要对一些突变进行过滤。如优先考虑蛋白中已知疾病基因的突变、根据医学知识确定优先级等。

Variants may need to be prioritized in the analysis to determine their relevance to a disease. This requires variant filtering.

十三、医学解释　Medical explanation

生物信息学正在迅速成熟为一个强大的学科,然而当今生物信息学的方法远不能充分解释全基因组/全外显子组测序数据。因此,这些数据应该在医学背景下讨论。需要了解受试者的临床特征和相关的具体情况,最好是与其个人医生密切合作。如今推荐多学科的医生小组,将病理学家、生物信息学家、遗传学家、家庭医生、护师等医疗专业人员汇集在一起,讨论可能的变异及其临床相关性,给出诊断、护理的最佳建议。

Bioinformatics approaches do not explain adequately WES/WGS data. Therefore, these data should be discussed in the medical context. A multidisciplinary team of doctors is recommended for the discussion of potential variants or their clinical relevance. Therefore, the team can provide diagnosis, advice, and best care.

第四节 ◎ 遗传病的生物信息诊断、分析与咨询
Application of bioinformatics in genetic disease

姓名:马×　　性别:女　　出生日期:1992 年 03 月 24 日

民族:汉　　　地址:山西省××县××乡

就诊日期:2017 年 6 月 15 日

主诉:此前因视力低下就诊时发现:四肢细长,左右眼严重近视,二尖瓣关闭不全。医师提醒 Marfan 综合征的风险,但并未进一步检查。目前已怀孕 12 周,期待知道所怀胎儿是否正常。

Name: Ma　　Gender: Female　　Date of Birth: March 24,1992

Address: ×× County, ×× Town, Shanxi Province

Date of visit: June 15,2017

Chief complaint: Ms. Ma has slender limbs and severe myopia in both eyes. She has mitral regurgitation. A physician has warned her of the risk of Marfan syndrome. At present, Ms. Ma has been pregnant for 12 weeks and she is anxious to learn if her unborn baby is healthy.

一、诊断

(一) 马×的诊断

1. 病史与家族史采集

患者马×,27 岁,病史见主诉;无家族史。

2. 症状与体征

身材高挑、四肢细长,拇指长过掌宽。手指环绕腕部时超过一圈。双眼严重近视达 900 度,晶状体半脱位。脊柱侧凸达 20°。二尖瓣关闭不全。

初步诊断:根据患者的症状与体征,初步判断可能为 Marfan 综合征,须进一步检查以确诊。

Physical Symptoms: Slender limbs; Joint hypermobility; and Aracnodactyly (Steinberg sign and Walter-Murdoch sign); Severe myopia in both eyes up to 9.0 diopters; Lens dislocation; Scoliosis; Mitral regurgitation.

According to the symptoms and the physical characteristics, Ms. Ma was suspected of having Marfan syndrome.

3. 遗传学全外显子组检查

考虑便捷性及患者的经济能力,采用全外显子组检查(见本节附录)。患者外周静脉采血 5 ml,肝素抗凝,冻存后送检。(详见后附实验)

检查结果:患者 NM_000138.4:c.4205G＞A;NP_000129.3:p.Cys1402Tyr;发生错义突变。ClinVar 检测结果显示为有害突变。有两篇文献(PMID:11748851,PMID:17657824)证实此突变的患者具有心血管病的表型。

生物信息学给出参考意见:考虑 Marfan 综合征。

医师诊断:综合生物信息学参考意见和临床指征,考虑为 Marfan 综合征。Marfan 综合征为常染色体显性遗传病,胎儿有可能也患有 Marfan 综合征。由于其心血管病风险,患者需密切观察怀孕期间的心血管指标。为明确突变来源,患者直系家属也应进行相关检查。

Diagnosis:The combination of physical symptoms with genetic analysis led to a diagnosis of Marfan syndrome. It was suggested that the cardiovascular indicators of Ms. Ma be observed closely during pregnancy.

(二)马×的产前诊断

1. 病史

初次妊娠,目前孕 12 周,无明显早孕反应,孕前和孕后均无患病、服药和接触有害物质。在当地医院做产前检查均正常。

2. 胎儿产前筛查

绒毛膜活检,全外显子组测序(见本节附录)。

检查结果:与马× 相同,送检者 NM_000138.4:c.4205G＞A;NP_000129.3:p.Cys1402Tyr;发生错义突变。ClinVar 检测结果显示为有害突变。有两篇文献(PMID:11748851,PMID:17657824)证实此突变的患者具有心血管病的表型。

生物信息学给出参考意见:考虑 Marfan 综合征。

产前诊断:由于仅有生物信息学指标,判断胎儿可能具有 Marfan 综合征,需密切观察。出生后应持续监测至成年期。

Diagnosis:based on genetic analysis,prenatal diagnosis indicates that the fetus may have Marfan syndrome. It was suggested that the indicators of Marfan syndrome be observed closely in the child.

二、遗传咨询与治疗

对马×和胎儿已作明确诊断,该疾病为常染色体显性遗传病,根据该病的性质、发病原理等特点,给予相应的遗传咨询。

(一)对策和措施

1. 告知与解释

向马×解释诊断结果和产前诊断结果,告知该病的症状、原理、预后等情况,使其对 Marfan 综合征有充分的了解。

The results of her diagnosis and the prenatal diagnosis were explained to Ms.

Ma. She was informed of the symptoms，principles，and prognosis；therefore，Ms. Ma has a good understanding of Marfan syndrome.

2. 建议和措施

因胎儿确诊为 Marfan 综合征,有理由施行人工流产。但应由患者及其伴侣自行做出决定,咨询医师不应替他们做出决定。

在 Marfan 综合征患者的妊娠晚期,主动脉夹层风险增加。可能导致孕产妇死亡和胎儿死亡。马×主动脉直径尚未发生扩张,妊娠风险较低。应由患者及其伴侣自行做出决定。

建议如考虑再度怀孕的话,应再次作孕前诊断。怀孕前应考虑预防性主动脉手术。

The fetus was diagnosed with Marfan syndrome. The diameter of the aorta has not yet expanded so the risk of the pregnancy is low. The couple should reach their own decisions regarding artificial abortion.

Pre-pregnancy diagnosis or prophylactic aortic surgery should be considered before pregnancy.

（二）Marfan 综合征的治疗

1. 持续监测

为控制主动脉疾病,对 Marfan 综合征患者应进行持续超声监测。当主动脉直径稳定时,可以每年监测一次。若有不稳定情况应遵医嘱监测。

对于其直系亲属也应该进行 Marfan 综合征的评估。

All patients with Marfan syndrome should undergo an echocardiographic monitoring annually. Patients who show aortic dilatation should be checked more frequently.

2. 药物及手术治疗

使用 β 受体阻滞剂等药物可能减缓 Marfan 综合征的心血管风险。进行主动脉预防性手术可能最大限度改善 Marfan 综合征的心血管症状。术后仍需进行检测和 β 受体阻滞剂等药物的治疗。二尖瓣脱垂的患者应考虑手术修复。这是首选的治疗方案。

β-blockers reduce aortic wall stress because of their inotropic and negative chronotropic effects. While prophylactic surgery on the aortic root has the greatest impact on the survival of patients with Marfan syndrome, mitral valve prolapse is common in patients with this syndrome. Surgical repair of mitral valve prolapse is always the preferred treatment option，if technically feasible.

3. 生活方式改变

生活中应关注个人心血管情况。运动时应考虑个人的心血管状态。应制定系统性和渐进的运动计划。避免短跑等爆发性运动。避免举重等强烈的静态运动。运动时心率不应大于每分钟 100 次。非竞技性的运动如游泳、慢跑等比较推荐。

Physical exercise contributes to the progressive dilatation of the aortic root. Non-competitive sports with a constant level of activity，such as swimming or jogging，are preferable.

4. 怀孕相关问题

Marfan 综合征是常染色体显性遗传病。有近 50% 的概率传递给后代。想要生孩子的患者应该在孕前接受遗传咨询。伴侣中一人患有 Marfan 综合征的可以利用体外受精、胚胎植入前诊断等辅助生殖方法。怀孕期间可以进行产前诊断。胎儿若受到影响，可以考虑人工流产。

Couples with one affected partner can choose assisted reproduction therapy to avoid transmitting the disease to their children.

5. 产妇相关问题

妊娠期间心血管会发生大量变化。心率和收缩期容积在妊娠期间均增加。另外，激素变化可影响主动脉壁变化。当患者已有严重的瓣膜反流时，妊娠可能导致心衰。妊娠期间主动脉夹层风险增大。妊娠期间发生主动脉夹层与 50% 的产妇死亡相关。有报道指出若没有发生主动脉扩张的现象，妊娠风险可控。并且可选择阴道分娩。欧洲心脏病学会推荐，主动脉根部直径＜40 mm 可以妊娠。若主动脉直径≥40 mm 建议首先进行主动脉置换术。最终的决定应该适合个人。医师应该根据患者个人情况综合考虑，并向患者详细解释妊娠风险。

Some guidelines discourage patients with Marfan syndrome from becoming pregnant. According to the European Society of Cardiology，for patients with an aortic root diameter ＜40 mm，pregnancy is not normally contraindicated. For patients with an aortic root diameter ≥40 mm，elective aortic replacement surgery is recommended. The physician should consider the patient's individual circumstances and explain the pregnancy risk to the patient in detail.

（三）随访

对咨询者进行随访，了解咨询的结果，特别是对马×是否选择人工流产、是否考虑再次受孕进行随访，以便给予进一步的咨询。

The couple should discuss the options described above and reach a decision regarding whether they should discontinue the pregnancy. Follow-up should be conducted to understand the results of the consultation.

三、附录 Appendix

病例相关生物信息学分析：全外显子组生物信息学分析步骤流程如图 13-3 所示。

患者样本送达后，使用标准试剂盒提取基因组 DNA，捕获试剂盒富集外显子区，经 Illumina 测序仪测序后获得 BCL 文件，使用 bcl2fastq2 软件将其转换为可操作的 *. fastq. gz 文件。为简单起见，这里给出两个简化版本。命名为 test_R1. fastq. gz，test_R2. fastq. gz。我们以此为例进行简单的生物信息学运算。

1. 运算环境准备 Computing environment preparation

由于 GATK 分析软件需要 POSIX 操作系统，可以使用 Linux、MacOSX 等系统进行工作。使用 GAT 前需要安装 JAVA 环境。可以使用 GATK 下载地址：https：//software. broadinstitute. org/gatk/。除此之外，还需要下载 BWA 软件包。地址：http：//bio-bwa. sourceforge. net/。本实验所需的各类软件及测序结果文件下载地址：http：//medicine. fudan. eda. cn/genetics/down. aspx？ info_lb＝672&flag＝101。

推荐使用 bioconda（https：//bioconda. github. io/）进行运算环境配置和软件安装，详细操作可以参考 https：//bioconda. github. io/页面的说明。

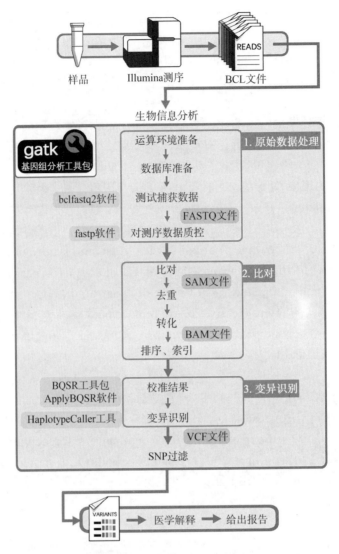

图 13-3   生物信息学分析简要流程

Fig. 13-3   Bioinformatics workflows

The GATK analysis software requires the POSIX operating system. A JAVA environment is also required. The GATK and BWA package can be freely downloaded.

2. 数据库准备   Reference genome preparation

从这里下载 hg19 基因组序列:http://hgdownload. soe. ucsc. edu/goldenPath/hg19/bigZips/hg19.2bit,请注意下载到的序列是二进制格式,需要转化为 fasta 格式。使用 twoBitToFa 软件转换格式,可在 http://hgdownload. cse. ucsc. edu/admin/exe/linux. x86_64/下载。

twoBitToFa hg19.2bit hg19. fa(对二进制文件进行格式转换)

bwa index hg19. fa(使用 BWA 等对数据库索引,方便后续比对及变异分析)

samtools faidx hg19. fa

../src/gatk-4.0.11.0/gatk CreateSequenceDictionary

-R ../db/hg19.fa

-O ../db/hg19.dict

经过索引之后的文件列表如图 13－4 所示。

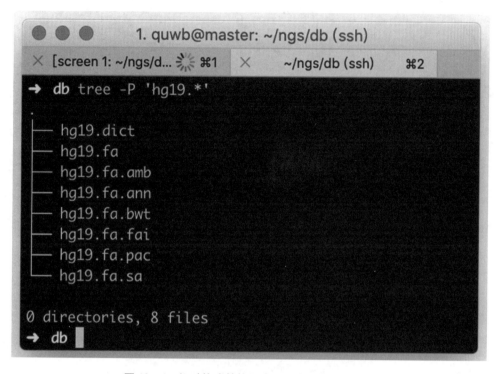

图 13－4 经过格式转换及索引的参考基因组文件
Fig. 13－4 Indexing reference genome FASTA files

3. 测试捕获数据 Test the capture data

test_R1.fastq.gz

test_R2.fastq.gz

4. 使用 fastp 对测序数据质控,fastp 的功能类似于 fastqc＋Trimmomatic,使用简单且速度较快(图 13－5,图 13－6) FASTP is used for quality control of the sequencing data (Fig. 13－5,Fig. 13－6)

fastp

-w 16(使用 16 线程进行计算,线程数越多,速度越快,决定于计算服务器的 CPU)

-i test_R1.fastq.gz

-I test_R2.fastq.gz

-o test_R1.clean.fastq.gz

-O test_R2.clean.fastq.gz

(fastp 除生成两个经过过滤后的 clean 数据之外,还生成了两个格式不同的质控报告,html 方便研究者阅读,json 格式方便后续脚本解析。html 报告详细地列出了质控前后数据的统计信息。)

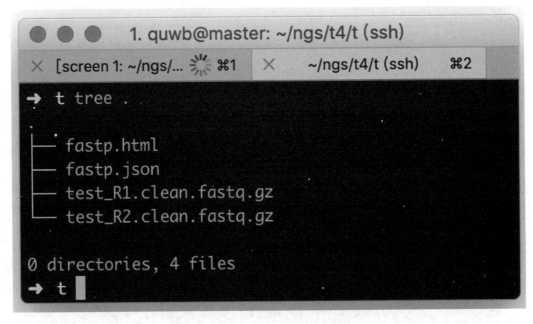

图 13 - 5　经过质控过滤后的测序文件

Fig. 13 - 5　QC-filtered sequencing files

fastp report

Summary

General

fastp version:	0.19.5 (https://github.com/OpenGene/fastp)
sequencing:	paired end (125 cycles + 125 cycles)
mean length before filtering:	125bp, 125bp
mean length after filtering:	122bp, 122bp
duplication rate:	11.776433%
Insert size peak:	139

Before filtering

total reads:	677.144000 K
total bases:	84.643000 M
Q20 bases:	78.001854 M (92.153934%)
Q30 bases:	71.630793 M (84.626954%)
GC content:	45.811511%

After filtering

total reads:	654.640000 K
total bases:	80.226878 M
Q20 bases:	74.915253 M (93.379245%)
Q30 bases:	69.381422 M (86.481518%)

图 13 - 6　质控报告

Fig. 13 - 6　Quality control report

5. 比对,得到 SAM 文件　Alignment. Output the SAM file

../src/bwa mem

-t 16

-R'@RG\tID:CKD518452\tPL:illumina\tLB:WES\tSM:test'

../db/hg19.fa

test_R1.clean.fastq.gz

test_R2.clean.fastq.gz

＞ test.align.sam

6. 对该 SAM 文件去重　Use samblaster for deduplication of the SAM file

../src/samblaster

-i test.align.sam

-o test.dedup.sam

7. 将 SAM 转化成 BAM 格式　Format conversion:from SAM to BAM

samtools view -b -S test.dedup.sam＞test.dedup.bam

8. 对 BAM 文件进行排序　Sort BAM files

samtools sort test.dedup.bam -f test.dedup.sorted.bam

9. 对 BAM 进行索引　Index BAM files

samtools index test.dedup.sorted.bam

10. 使用 BQSR(Recalibration Base Quality Score)工具包重新校准结果　Recalibrate the results using the Base Quality Score Recalibration(BQSR)kit. This step requires the VCF file for the annotation site.

这一步骤需要先下载 BQSR 需要的注释位点 VCF 文件。该文件可在 ftp://gsapubftp-anonymous @ ftp.broadinstitute.org/bundle/hg19/下载:1000G_phase1.snps.high_confidence.hg19.sites.vcf.gz

1000G_phase1.indels.hg19.sites.vcf.gz。运行 BQSR,先使用 BaseRecalibrator 命令生成一个 recal.data.table 中间文件:

../src/gatk-4.0.11.0/gatk

--java-options "-Xmx32G" BaseRecalibrator

-R ../db/hg19.fa

-I test.dedup.sorted.bam

-O recal_data.table

--known-sites ../db/1000G_phase1.snps.high_confidence.hg19.sites.vcf.gz

--known-sites ../db/1000G_phase1.indels.hg19.sites.vcf.gz

11. 再运行 ApplyBQSR 校准　Run the ApplyBQSR calibration again.

../src/gatk-4.0.11.0/gatk

--java-options "-Xmx32G" ApplyBQSR

-R ../db/hg19.fa

-I test.dedup.sorted.bam

--bqsr-recal-file recal_data. table

-O test. dedup. sorted. BQSR. bam

12. 变异识别 Mutation recognition

获得新的 BAM 文件后，使用 HaplotypeCaller 工具对上述的 BAM 文件进行变异识别，生成一个 VCF 文件，用于后续位点的质控和注释，最简单的单样本变异识别如下，从一个 bam 到一个 vcf 文件(图 13 - 7)。

Variant calling is performed by HaplotypeCaller to generate a VCF file for quality control and annotation of the subsequent procedure.

../src/gatk-4.0.11.0/gatk

--java-options "-Xmx32G" HaplotypeCaller

-R ../db/hg19.fa -I test. dedup. sorted. BQSR. bam

--dbsnp ../db/1000G_phase1. snps. high_confidence. hg19. sites. vcf. gz

-O test. raw. vcf

vcf 文件可以用 Excel 软件打开，里面显示了变异的基因组坐标，变异前后的碱基差异等。

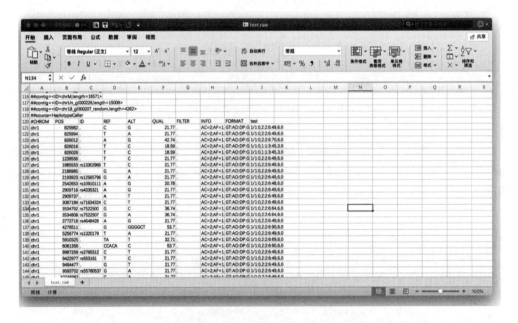

图 13 - 7 用 Excel 软件打开最终得到的 VCF 格式的变异识别文件
Fig. 13 - 7 The final VCF format variation recognition file opened with Excel software

获得的 test. raw. vcf 即是输出的经过计算的结果。对于真实测序数据，还需进一步的 SNP 过滤，并与 ClinVar 等数据库比对，找到关注的突变。并给出报告。

The obtained test. raw. vcf is the calculated output result. In clinical practice, further SNP filtering is needed. The output data need to be compared with databases such as ClinVar to identify the mutations of interest. The final report is given based on the calculations.

（杨云龙）

图书在版编目(CIP)数据

医学细胞与遗传学实验教程:汉英对照/杨玲,刘雯主编. —2 版. —上海:复旦大学出版社,
2020.8
ISBN 978-7-309-15145-9

Ⅰ.①医… Ⅱ.①杨… ②刘… Ⅲ.①医学-细胞生物学-实验-教材-汉、英 ②医学遗传学-实
验-教材-汉、英 Ⅳ.①R329.2-33 ②R394-33

中国版本图书馆 CIP 数据核字(2020)第 119224 号

医学细胞与遗传学实验教程:汉英对照(第二版)
杨　玲　刘　雯　主编
责任编辑/王　瀛

复旦大学出版社有限公司出版发行
上海市国权路 579 号　邮编:200433
网址:fupnet@ fudanpress.com　http://www.fudanpress.com
门市零售:86-21-65102580　　团体订购:86-21-65104505
外埠邮购:86-21-65642846　　出版部电话:86-21-65642845
杭州日报报业集团盛元印务有限公司

开本 787×1092　1/16　印张 13.5　字数 320 千
2020 年 8 月第 2 版第 1 次印刷

ISBN 978-7-309-15145-9/R·1825
定价:58.00 元

如有印装质量问题,请向复旦大学出版社有限公司出版部调换。
版权所有　　侵权必究